MARTIAL DANCE

Chaz Wilson
Pineapple Workshop
24th Sept.

D1741468

MARTIAL DANCE

total fitness with martial arts aerobics

Chaz Wilson

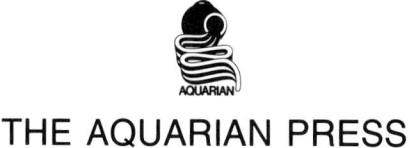

THE AQUARIAN PRESS

First published 1988

© Chaz Wilson 1988

All rights reserved. No part of this book may be reproduced or utilized in any form or by any means, electronic or mechanical, including photocopying, recording, or by an information storage and retrieval system, without permission in writing from the Publisher.

British Library Cataloguing in Publication Data

Wilson, Chaz.
Martial dance
1. Martial arts. Dancing
I. Title
796.8

ISBN 0-85030-758-9

The Aquarian Press is part of the Thorsons Publishing Group,
Wellingborough, Northamptonshire, NN8 2RQ, England

Typeset by MJL Limited, Hitchin, Hertfordshire
Printed in Great Britain by Woolnough Bookbinding Limited,
Irthlingborough, Northamptonshire

1 3 5 7 9 10 8 6 4 2

CONTENTS

INTRODUCTION

Martial dance is by definition **a form of dance utilizing martial arts techniques** which include kicks, strikes, punches, blocks and stances, and these movements are performed in different ways. Sometimes they are hard, fast and explosive, while at other times soft, slow and more fluid. From time to time the movements are performed slowly with muscle tensing, or frozen momentarily to hold a stance.

Martial dance can be appreciated at different levels. As an exercise it strengthens the body, improves coordination, balance, suppleness, and provides the added bonus of being artistic and therefore aesthetically gratifying. It can be practised for an hour or so, once or twice a week, or it can be perfected with dedication into an art form. Furthermore it can be used as self-defence training, although this is obviously not its primary aim nor its most practical function. Last, martial dance is a martial art and therefore a doorway to the philosophy and metaphysical principles that underlie the martial arts — or 'Budo' as they are collectively known.

Ultimately the purpose of martial dance, beyond its exercise and aesthetic value, is to act as a vehicle for meditation, a catalyst that brings the mind and the body into harmony. The ideas of self-improvement and self-awareness through athletic training are intrinsic to the martial arts. The philosophy of martial dance is that we must identify ourselves as warriors — that is, people who believe we must always show a fighting spirit in life — and that we can further reinforce this self image by performing martial dance. Martial dance is a way of saying — 'I am a fighting spirit'.

You can study martial dance for a lifetime — it will develop and hone your body and mind simultaneously, healing the rift that so often exists between the two. It is not only a hymn to the human body, it is a way of life that helps the practitioner relate to the meaning of existence and the world around us. Martial dance is the way of peace — the way of channelling the warrior spirit into a wider quest than combat expertise.

Both sexes will benefit equally from martial dance, as will martial artists and non martial artists. Martial dance is ideally suited to anyone who believes their body needs exercise and who appreciates the kinetic beauty of the martial arts. Because it does not have to involve sparring or physical combat, it can appeal to people of all temperaments and physical capabilities. The martial arts, hitherto, have been esoteric in the sense that the vast majority of mankind does not participate. Martial dance is potentially a mass communicator and can help to popularize and extend Budo's sphere of influence.

PART ONE
MARTIAL DANCE BACKGROUND

1

THE WAY OF PEACE

We live in a society that is growing increasingly apprehensive about the prevalence of crime and street violence. In the nocturnal sub-culture of discos, night clubs and pubs, excessive drinking increasingly leads to gratuitous violence. Censorship of the arts, especially television, is usually offered as a remedy but art is the innocent victim, the scapegoat of a society that has failed to properly educate its children. Aggression is something that needs to be harnessed and made to work for us not against us. The education system could substantially benefit from the precepts of etiquette and self-discipline that are inherent in the martial arts.

It is right that Budo should have both an aggressive and non-aggressive dimension. It must teach self-defence but also offer the hope of an alternative to meeting violence head-on with more violence. Meeting force with force is only a short-term remedy. In the long-term view the warrior must justify his existence as a person of peace as well as war; as a person who can apply all his martial spirit to the cause of peace and civilization.

HISTORICAL PRECEDENT FOR CONTEMPORARY MARTIAL DANCE

In a sense martial dance is as old as man himself. Men have always danced and they have always been warriors. Every primal war dance was a martial dance and there have been, through the ages, countless tribes and cultures with indigenous dances that celebrate and actually engender the martial spirit. Dance has always been used by man as a spiritual rocket fuel to propel himself into the realms of power or to invoke the gods

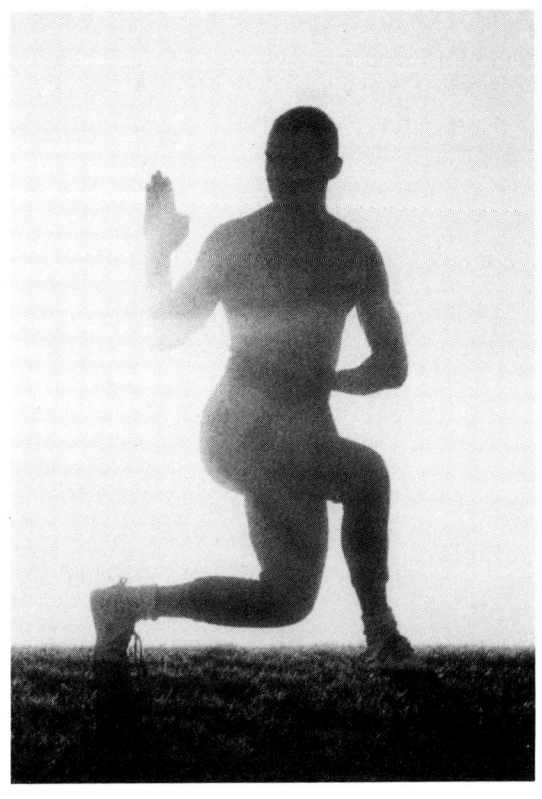

On television now we see what are
called 'beauty exercises' for women,
and I have thought watching them
how effectively our karate kata could be
utilized for this purpose, since they can
be practised everywhere.

Gichin Funakoshi
(Karate-do: My Way of Life)

even to the point of possession. But nearer home there are also precedents within the traditions of the martial arts.

Ram Muay

There is a centuries old tradition of dance in Thai Boxing called **Ram Muay** which literally means 'boxing dance'. It is similar to karate kata and kung fu in form. Each boxing camp has its own particular Ram Muay movements which incorporate all the basics of actual Thai Boxing and are performed to music. The dance takes place in the ring before the full contact fight begins, in full view of the opponent.

A typical dance might well begin with a fighter bowing three times while facing in the direction that he was born or alternatively the camp he belongs to. The movements are all symbolic — for example, outstretched hands pulling back in a drinking motion symbolize invoking the elements of Earth, Air, Fire, and Water to give him power and added confidence in his forthcoming fight. The fighter then picks up an imaginary spear and with his free hand points to the opposition's corner. He runs at his opponent and hurls the spear at him. This action has killed the adversary and the dancer picks up a make-believe spade and digs a hole or grave. He finishes his ritual by dragging the body across the ring and burying it, pushing the soil over the corpse and stamping it down.

Capoeira

In Brazil an indigenous martial art, known as **Capoeira**, was widespread at the dawn of the twentieth century. It is a combat training that encompasses dance and posits the existence of a force similar to the Chinese chi called 'axé', which is an internal power existing in nature — capable of being transmitted through specific rituals. In Capoeira, axé means the connection with roots, a special energy to be developed by any Capoeirista. As a dance it incorporates many martial techniques and even includes acrobatics. The music helps the student to develop physically while it enhances the awareness of the philosophical side of the art. In addition to the instrumental music, the chants are very important and the lyrics of the songs reflect many aspects of Brazilian life. Capoeira is therefore especially interesting for the martial dancer because it is a martial art that

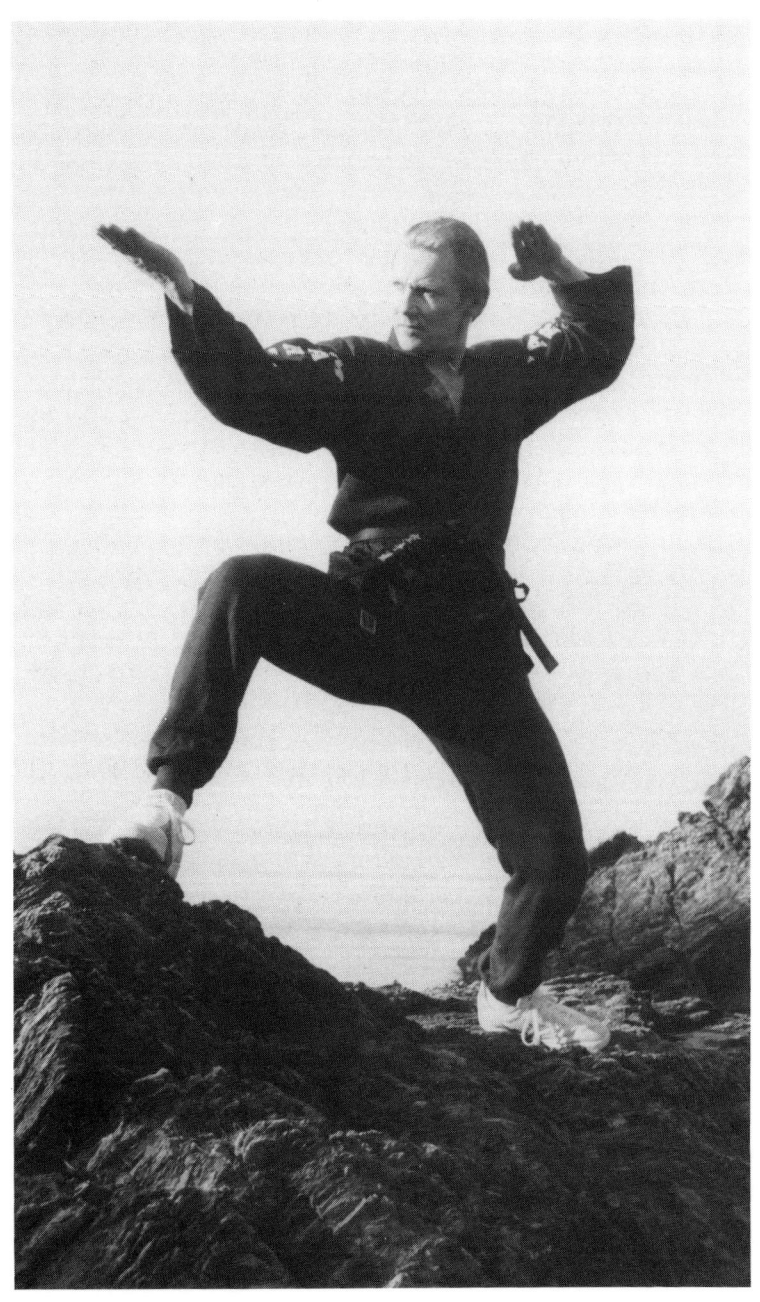

has developed its own special brand of music incorporating songs and chants that reflect the martial philosophy. Here we have an example of a martial art that, being a way of life, extends its sphere of influence to encompass other art forms which themselves serve the martial philosophy.

Wrestling

The interconnection between religion, dance and combat is further demonstrated in Turkey even to this day. **Wrestling** matches are preceded by ritualistic dance. When wrestlers meet for their open-air contests there is a warm-up ceremony called the 'pesrev' that goes beyond the sport into the realms of art and religion. The announcer begins his call to wrestling which is virtually a prayer, and then the drums commence.

The wrestlers, sometimes as many as 160 men in a line stretching across the arena, begin to strut in time with the drums, waving their hands and arms, moving forward, then backward. Then kneeling with their left knee on the ground, they move their right hand from the ground to the knee, lips, and forehead — a variant of the Muslim greeting of respect, touching hand to lips and brow — three times. There are also specific chants used to accompany the drum music.

Japanese Sumo wrestling is also impregnated with ceremony and religious ritual. The fighting area itself is blessed and can be said to function during the tournament as a religious shrine. Sumo has existed for centuries and is, of course, a popular sport today in Japan.

Wrestling also formed part of the 'pankration' — one of the earliest martial arts. It was practised by the Ancient Greeks and was a fusion of wrestling, boxing and kicking techniques. In passing it should be noted that the Greeks, who conceived the Olympic games, made sport into a religious festival, and there was even a war-dance called the 'pyrrhic', which is the nearest thing to a forerunner of the martial arts kata.

2

KATA

When a boxer shadow boxes, he is practising his techniques against an imaginary opponent. The **kata**, or form, is the martial arts equivalent to this, but because karate and kung fu have a much wider range of movements than pugilism, kata is a more elaborate and visually dynamic exercise. A kata, and there are hundreds of them in a range of styles, is a sequence of fighting techniques that have been formalized into a fixed solo routine that is learned by the martial artist and practised repeatedly until it becomes automatic. Many kata include a complex spectrum of movements incorporating kicks, strikes, punches, blocks, tension movements, spins and stances. Kata can be seen as a majestic solo war dance — but it is a war dance that is not so much about violence as about power. It is the warrior's dance of power.

There are some martial artists who emphasize the practical side of kata as a serious combat discipline, and there are others who see it more as an aesthetic experience or martial dance. Both points of view are justified but this thesis subscribes to the latter viewpoint and holds kata in essence to be a mystical exercise, a ritual that has more to do with the beauty of body movement and philosophical meditation than with self-defence. Whatever one's perspective, kata is excellent physical and mental training developing balance, focus of mind and body, coordination, fighting spirit, and many other attributes the martial artist needs to gain mastery of his body.

The self-defence aspect of Budo is only the base of the triangle, whereas its apex is character-perfection and enlightenment. The ultimate aim of training, in every martial art, should be the ideal of the spiritual warrior — a man or woman of wisdom whose physical power is merely a reflection of the more

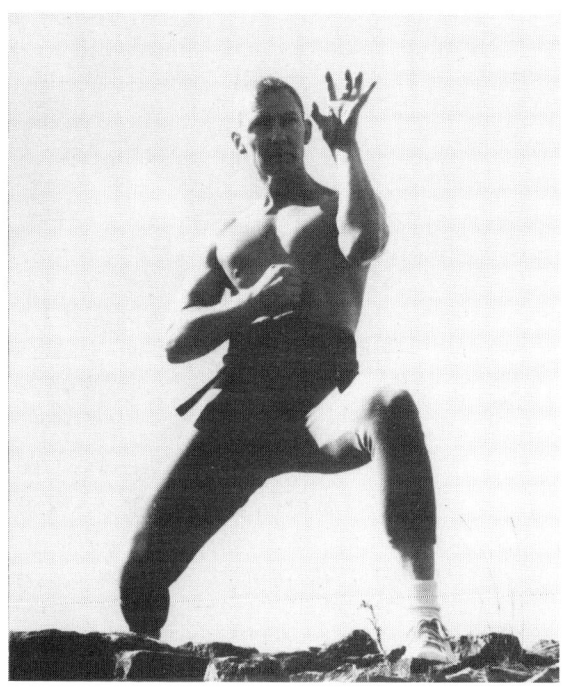

It is interesting that the dances of many peoples and races are linked with their representative boxing and jujutsu techniques. Iranian, Turkish, and Mongolian dancing and wrestling all show similarities. African native dancing and spear techniques are very similar. These similarities would be an interesting research topic.

Mas. Oyama
(This is Karate)

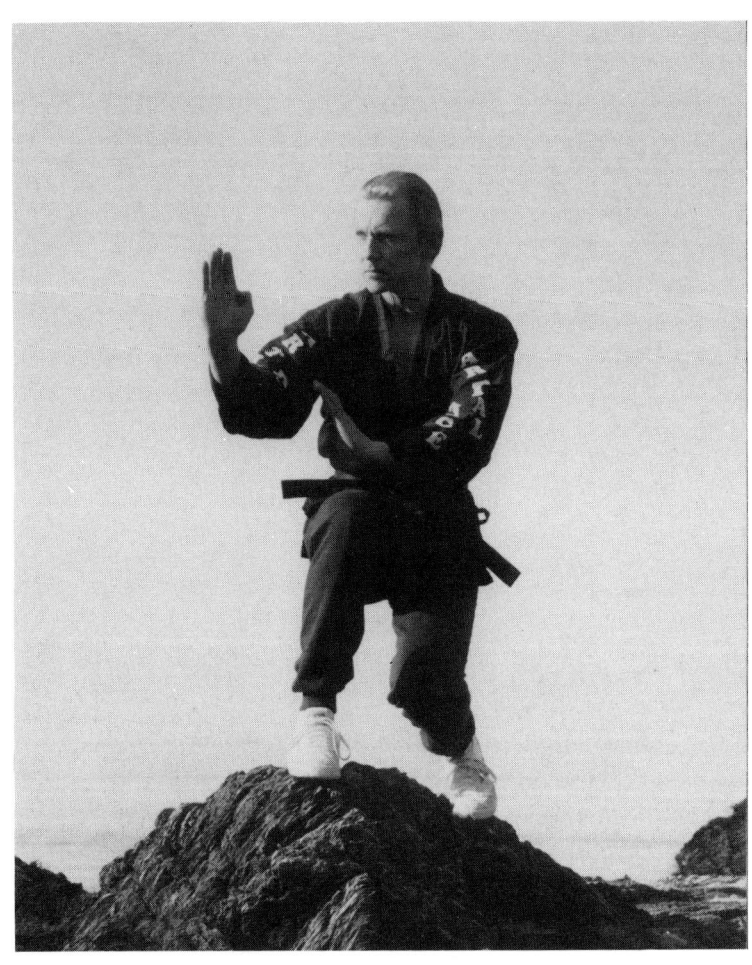

important power of the psyche. People do not have to be tough streetfighters or kickboxing champions to subscribe to the warrior philosophy, but it is important that they have some basic grasp of martial technique so that the body speaks the same language as the mind.

One trains in the martial arts not to get a black belt but a right mind. The mental approach, a perceptive grasp of the axioms of Budo, is more important than being a champion fighter. This is why martial dance is a road for everyone; it can give any able-bodied person a grounding in martial technique

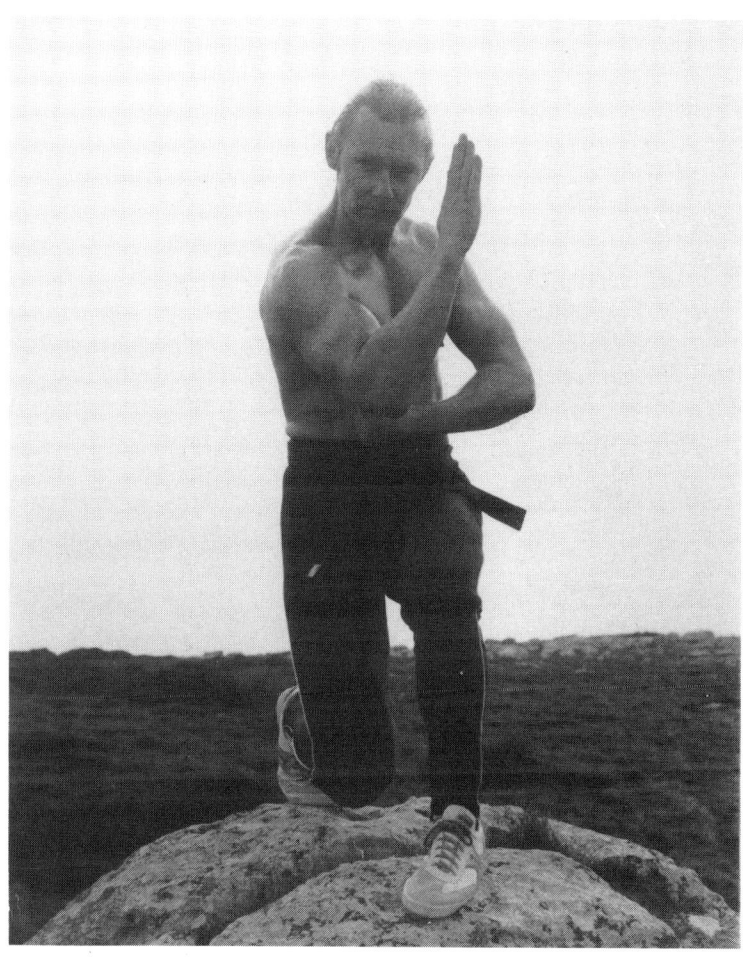

without making impractical demands on them physically. Not everyone has an equal appetite for physical training, especially where competitive fighting is concerned. Some only want to nibble, others to feast, but martial dance is a royal repast for all to enjoy according to their needs.

Martial dance is an extension of orthodox kata, a refinement of its dance potential. It is the logical progression from a proto-dance format to ritual or sacred dance — that is, dance that epitomizes the highest ideals of the spiritual warrior. Part of its beauty lies in the fact that it is unisex and egalitarian; men and women can participate on equal terms without the strength factor being relevant. The warrior movements are neither masculine nor feminine, but majestic expressions of kinetic power that symbolize the resilience of the human spirit, the fighting spirit of man and woman. Martial dance transcends violence and lifts Budo beyond the realm of banal physical combat, and it is the key to the universalization of the warrior ethic.

Martial dance building blocks are kata, and the martial dancer has artistic licence to destroy in order to create — or recreate. Every kata and form is at his disposal. Since the kata's inherent logic in terms of self-defence is less important to him than its aesthetic power and visual appeal, he is free to dismantle kata and reassemble them to suit his own dance-orientated arrangements and choreography. Taking from different styles, his eclectic appetite knows no bounds as he synthesizes the rounded flowing movements of kung fu with the harder more linear movements of karate. All stylistic boundaries are sacrificed to aesthetics.

Music greatly enhances martial dance, but it is not essential. The dance fits equally well with the sound of nature — with the music of the waterfall, the wind, and the birds. It can be performed in unison with others or alone on a hilltop. Anyone can do it, and by doing so they manifest their affirmation of the warrior credo.

3

FORMS AS A WAY OF SELF-ENLIGHTENMENT

Tai Chi Chuan is a Chinese martial art, and, although it is not strictly speaking a dance, it puts a great emphasis on the practise of forms and it is one of the least aggressive and most spiritual of all the martial arts. It therefore represents a fusion of spiritual culture with physical culture.

Martial dance in its highest form is a way to enlightenment, and this is true of Tai Chi Chuan. Tai Chi itself is the Grand Ultimate. It is the beginning and the end. It is the timeless, the infinite, the eternal, or if you prefer it is reality, truth or God. Chuan literally means fist but stands for the total physical man. The practise of Tai Chi Chuan is the practise of a complete physical culture and its purpose is to use Chuan as a vehicle for experiencing Tai Chi, the Grand Ultimate.

Tai Chi Chuan emphasizes the inward movement of the mind toward tranquillity and meditation. Vital force, known as 'Chi', is developed by breathing techniques, and soft, flowing forms which resemble a mystical dance. Concentration on the movement and flow of breathing is said to bring biorhythms of the body into harmony, integrating body and mind. This harmony relaxes the psychophysical unity and brings peace.

Tai Chi Chuan is both meditation and self-defence. The goal for the student is to be able to defend himself competently and efficiently according to the principle of softness upon which the system is based. Chi brings health and enlightenment but unless the movements or forms are practised properly, the cultivation of Chi is not possible. Chi is energy and this energy is power — Tai Chi Chuan movements are a dance of power.

The continuous movement of the forms without change in tempo or rhythm symbolizes the continuous flow of life. The beauty of Tai Chi Chuan does not lie in any particular form or

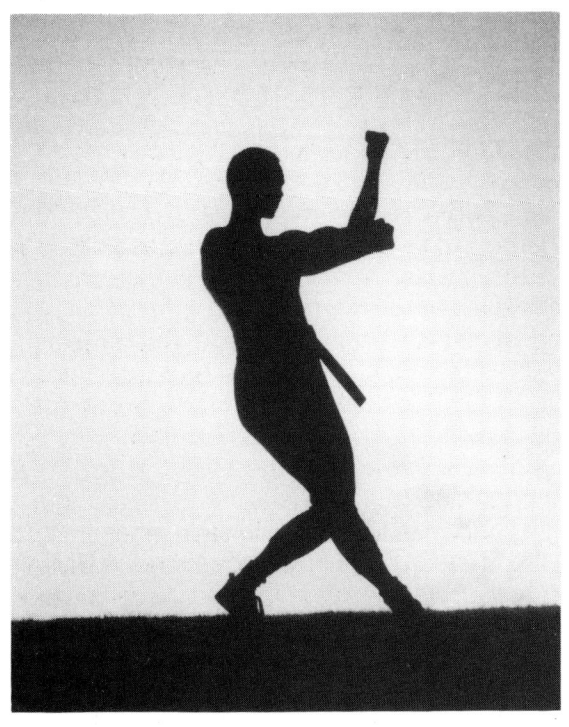

I often tell my young colleagues that no one can attain perfection in karate-do until he finally comes to realize that it is, above all else, a faith, a way of life. . . In as much as karate-do aims at perfection of mind as well as body, expressions that extol only physical prowess should never be used in connection with it.

Gichin Funakoshi
(Karate-do)

movement, but in the action of the whole spectrum of movements from beginning to end. The beauty of life lies not in any of its stages, but in the whole continuum from birth to death.

Kung Fu forms are often based on animals. This establishes an important principle, for by doing this the martial artist is showing himself to be studying nature and expressing his observations and conclusions in his art. These warriors attempted to discern and understand the fighting style of numerous animals, insects and birds, including praying mantis, hawk, eagle, swallow, monkey, and bear. They did not necessarily copy the movements exactly but tried to discover the meaning behind them and translate it into human movement. In this way they attuned their bodies to nature.

In **Hsing-i**, students are taught five fundamental postures, each one corresponding to one of the basic elements of fire, metal, wood, earth and water. In this way hsing-i goes past the study and imitation of nature in its animal forms to a celebration of the fundamental constituents of reality. If training has these philosophical connections, the mind and the body are exercised together, in harmony with each other and with nature.

Much the same approach is to be found in **Ninja** postures and hand poses. In ninjutsu there is a power-generating system based on the mystical idea of redirecting the intrinsic energy of nature through the hands. In this system each hand and finger symbolizes a specific attribute of the body's make-up. The hand poses are accompanied by specific chants. Each hand pose has its own chant which calls upon a particular personification of some aspect or deity for assistance in directing power. Likewise, the postures or stances correspond to the elemental manifestations of earth, water, fire and wind, and these determine different ways of fighting and dealing with an opponent.

In some styles, like **Pa-kua**, the forms enact the elemental dramas of creation and destruction in the world. In one form the movements are meant to symbolize the cosmic beginning of the Tao, the splitting of the cosmos into the elemental gender forces of yin and yang, and the resultant birth of the evolutionary process. The whole universe is seen to be governed by the tension of a sexual polarity, a male and female division which is represented by the movements of a martial artist in

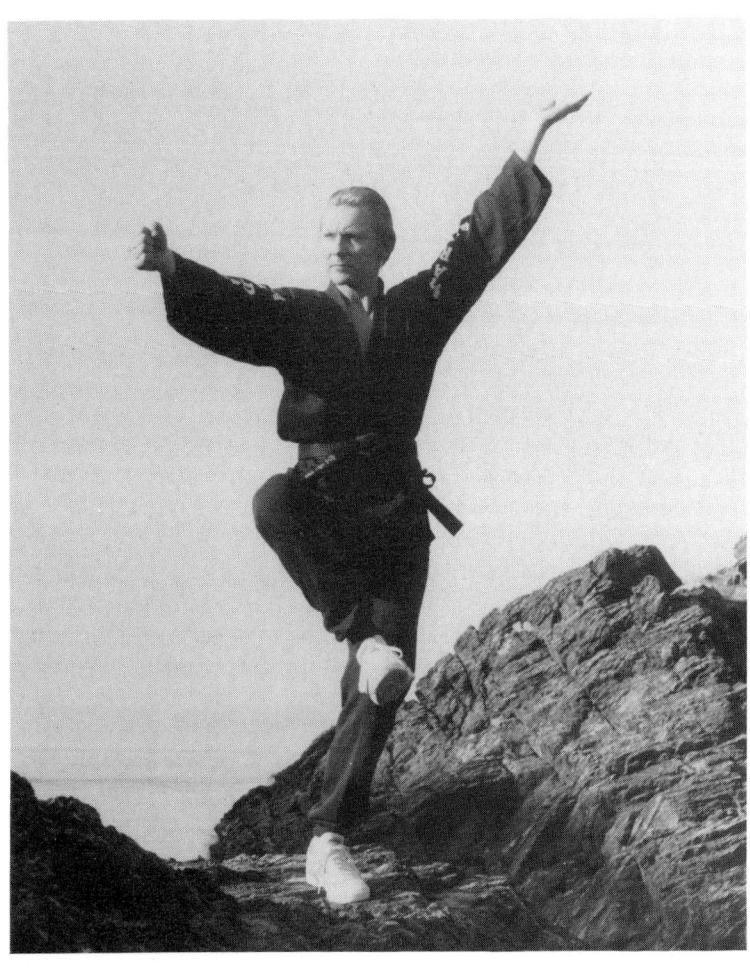

his power dance — the dance of truth which puts him in touch with his vision of life.

Here then we have a tradition of martial artists ingesting the awesome mysteries and miracles of nature and reflecting them in their physical and mental motions. Just as an artist or painter will be awestruck by the beauty of nature and will attempt to imitate it and celebrate it on a canvas, so the warrior recreates nature in his power dance. Without this anchorage in the natural world, without this profound liason with reality, kata and martial dance would be merely a technical exercise.

4

DYNAMIC TENSION

Sometimes in kata there are tension movements in which the muscles are flexed as the breath is exhaled. Such movements are closely related to dynamic tension exercises, isometrics and bodybuilding posing routines.

In **dynamic tension** one's muscles gain strength by working against other muscles in one's own body instead of against weights. Isometric exercises are similar but emphasize static exercises so that the muscles strain against an immovable resistance. In dynamic tension all exercises are performed with movement, sometimes performing free tension movements, sometimes using ones own body as a resistance. When a bodybuilder hits a posing routine he is utilizing both dynamic tension and isometrics. He is artistically tensing and flexing into poses which he holds for the sole purpose of making his muscles stand out. Thus he projects from his being an aura of power.

This form of exercise tones up the muscles and even develops strength, but its primary function in martial dance is to enhance visual impact. These tension movements look majestic and powerful, especially if the practitioner has muscular definition. Added to this, such movements are excellent for inducing kinesthetic awareness. Dynamic tension imparts a body awareness of each muscle, one focuses the mind on one's physicality with an intensity that doesn't exist in normal daily activities. Kinesthetic awareness is the awareness of muscles and tendons working off the skeleton, and this augmented body-consciousness extends to breathing.

We take breathing for granted of course, but without it we would die. We breathe in and out the air of life. The Chinese term for air is Chi — which is also an aspect of the life force.

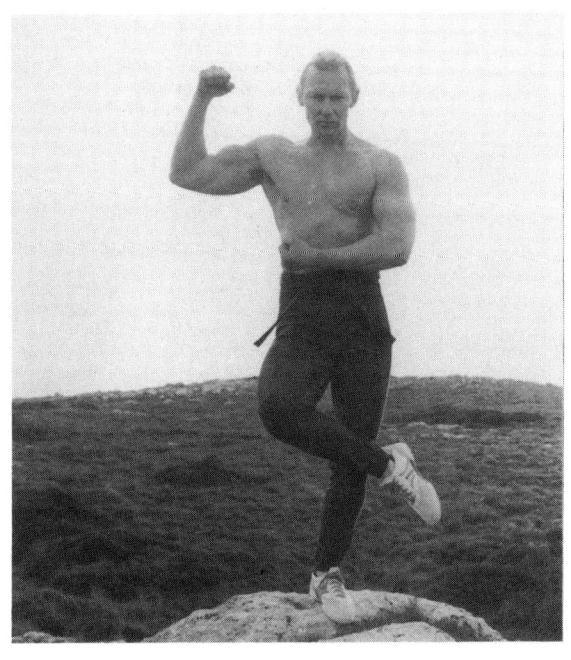

As soon as I began posing, I got a thundering applause from the British audience. What I was doing now was mostly for exhibition and my routine became ballet.

Arnold Schwarzenegger
(Winner of Mr Universe title, 1967)

Posing is muscle in motion. Every pose has got to flex. Every move you make should be for a reason.

Corrina Everson

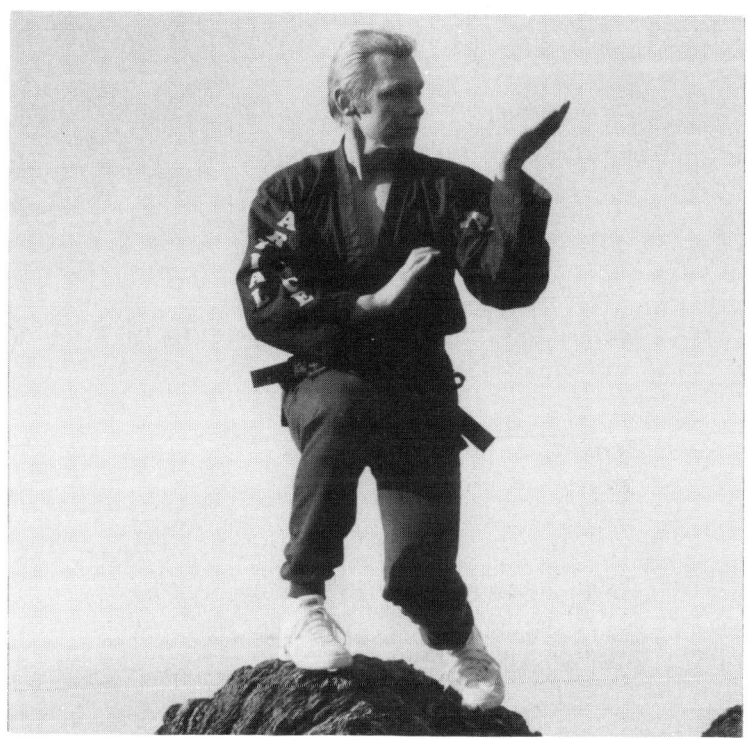

Proper breathing should be coordinated with all movements and is especially important in tension movements whereby the air is inhaled through the nose and exhaled audibly through the mouth.

Bodybuilders compete by a kind of dance of power similar to kata. They unwind a series of dramatic poses, sometimes twenty or more, and as each one is hit and held for a few seconds it is intended to convey a sense of awesome power and symmetry. One pose flows into another — the arms, legs, chest, back and midriff all flexed with a sharp intensity born of hours of relentless practice. Many of the poses resemble karate and kung fu stances, and the posing routines are always performed to music. One does not have to have a bodybuilder's build to carry them off, for they are aesthetically striking in themselves, although a few muscles in the right places will obviously help. Since martial dance is also a dance of power, it is greatly enriched with the adoption of poses from the bodybuilder's repertoire. These are then easily fused with dynamic tension movements to make an exciting kinetic vocabulary. Bodybuilders remind us that the human body can be a living sculpture.

The ancient Greeks, who invented the concept of the nude in art and began the Olympic Games, conceived of their gods and goddesses as perfectly formed humans because no amount of human imagination can conjure up anything more beautiful. The martial dancer should never forget that the human body is the masterpiece of natural evolution.

5

WEIGHT TRAINING/ BODYBUILDING

Bodybuilding, once a male preserve, is now practised by women who have achieved results that would have once been deemed impossible. The martial dancer should, ideally, train regularly with weights.

Although there is no sharp line of division between weight training and bodybuilding, the former tends to be about resistance exercises using free weights and machines to improve the functional strength of a muscle or muscle group and to develop muscle tone and definition. Bodybuilding is more cosmetic and aesthetic and is the process of shaping the body by the use of weight training and other disciplines for the sake of appearance. It is therefore a visual art/sport that uses progressive resistance exercises to build, tone, shape and define the muscles.

Many people are still repelled by the idea of lifting weights because they fear (wrongly) that they will get over-muscled like the champions that emblazon the pages of muscle magazines. These exemplars of their sport are not only pumping-iron fanatics but have unusual genetic gifts that enable them to make almost superhuman gains in muscle mass. As it happens, many of them are good all-round athletes and are surprisingly supple, but the martial dancer does not necessarily need this degree of muscularity.

Training with weights can only improve the appearance of the body, and this is important for the martial dancer because martial dance is not only about the craft of human movement, but about the beauty of the body itself. Female bodybuilders are not nearly as big as the men, but their balletic posing is often better than their male counterparts. The art of muscle in motion, of being a kinetic sculpture, is about the art of mov-

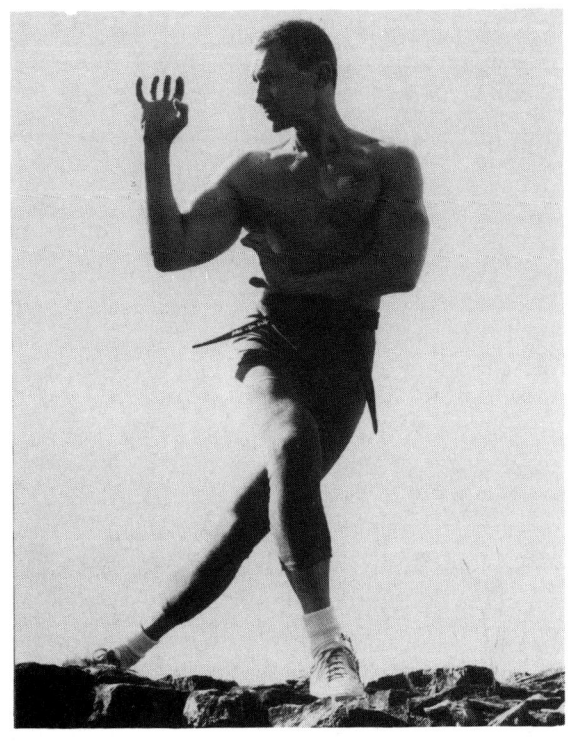

There can be no fairer spectacle than that of a man who combines the possession of moral goodness in his soul with the outward beauty of his body; corresponding and harmonizing with the former because the same great pattern enters into both if a man is eventually to achieve his high destiny.

Plato

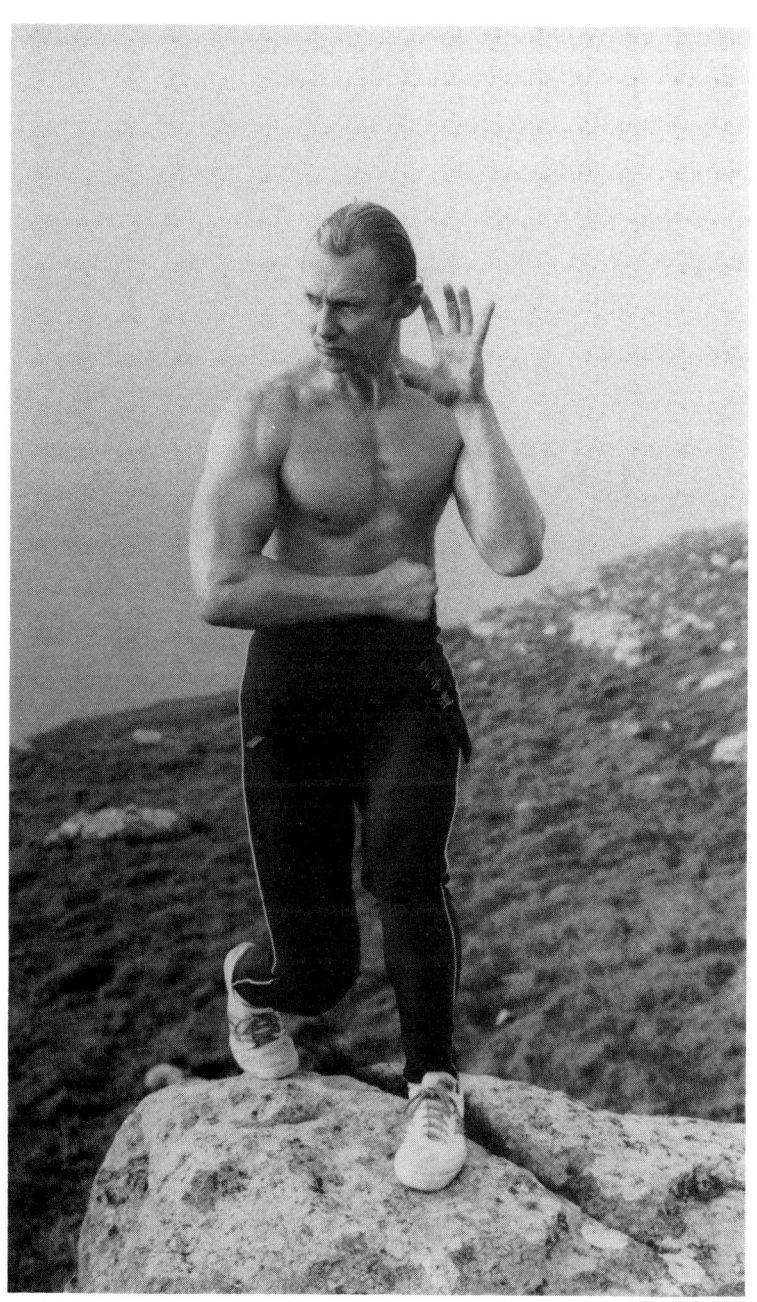

ing with power and majesty rather than body size.

Training with weights can reshape the body to a considerable extent and certainly improve everyone's physique or figure no matter what body type they are born with. And it is right that people should take a pride in their bodies and make the most of what they have got. Few people ever achieve the appearance they want, but it does no harm to have an ideal in one's mind's eye to which one can aspire.

At the end of the day, of course, we must not get too self-conscious about our looks. The aesthetic charisma of the young, fit, symmetrical body is only one side of the coin, and ultimately it must take a back seat to physiology. We all have bodies and whether by society's standards they are beautiful or not we are all living, breathing, fully-functioning miracles of natural engineering. We must take pride in this, and getting in shape is just the icing on the cake. Regular workouts in the gym will help us to present this complex cellular masterpiece to ourselves and to the world with more confidence and panache.

Using weights is very much a science, that is to say, there are simple laws of cause and effect that give the ability to predict results from chosen training techniques. This means that *you* are in control. The achievement of bulk is extremely difficult and is dependent on a whole range of factors that have to be right. There is no danger of over-development for the martial dancer who trains in moderation, and even quite heavy weights can be used to enhance the body's power. Two or three one-hour workouts per week are quite sufficient — even one will help, and in each session the whole body can be worked if you stick to the basic exercises.

6

THE MARTIAL DANCE LESSON

THE BOW

The martial dance lesson should be a full physical and mental workout. It begins and ends with a bow which symbolizes the mutual respect between students and teacher. It also gives the lesson a precise beginning and end — a precision and focus like the martial arts movements themselves. The bow is a sign of respect for the art of martial dance and a gesture of acknowledgement that as a student you are privileged to be learning it and are going to take your training seriously. The teacher is also privileged to be teaching and to have the opportunity to improve the world in his own small and humble way by passing on a knowledge system that is going to help people to improve themselves physically and mentally.

WARM-UPS AND STRETCHING

Warm-ups and stretching exercises can be found in martial arts clubs nationwide. They are performed to avoid injury by warning the muscles and joints of the imminent demands that are about to be placed upon them and also to warm up the heart and lungs. There are few things in life more frustrating for the serious student of physical culture than an injury, especially if it could have been easily avoided with a little preparatory attention to warm-ups. Being safety conscious is very important, but we cannot afford to get over-concerned or we would stop training altogether. For the dancer or athlete, over-use injuries are an occupational hazard and almost no one is spared altogether from injury during their years of training.

In martial dance, repetitions of techniques are probably more

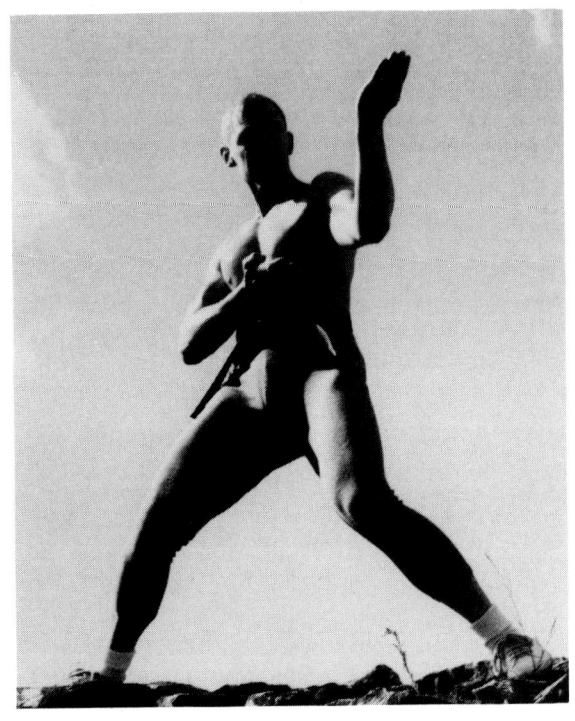

To be deadly serious is not just an essential for a follower of karate-do; it is equally essential in everyone's daily life, for life is itself a struggle to survive. Anyone so complacent as to assume that after a failure he will have another opportunity will seldom make much of a success of his life.

Gichin Funakoshi
(Karate-do)

numerous than in many traditional martial arts and if one trains daily it puts stress on vulnerable areas of the body such as the knees which are used a great deal in kicking. The movements of martial dance, especially the kicks, must have focus and power, but they do not have to be performed with full-blast effort and aggression because the rhythms of dance are more relaxed and continuous. In this way stress on the joints is minimized.

BASICS

After the body has been stretched and the muscles and joints warmed up, work can begin on **basic technique**. Basic does not mean only simple beginner's techniques, as the whole range of martial movements is open to selection and thus any kicks, punches, strikes, blocks, stances, tension postures or multiples might be chosen for detailed analysis.

Multiples entail performing several kicks with the same leg without putting the foot down between or, alternatively, several hand movements in quick succession. The hand multiples can be performed very fast and are not only good training for self-defence, developing speed and dexterity, but look impressive for their stark contrast to tension movements and the soft flowing motions. Multiples are advanced techniques, as are jumping and spinning kicks. These are covered in this section because basics covers any technique that can be used as a unit — a 'basic' building block in martial dance choreography. Even advanced techniques can be made quite simple if they are broken down for the student into easy manageable stages. The idea of basics is to take the techniques individually before they are amalgamated and built up into routines and sequences. In this way their main characteristics can be practised and their finer points of detail analysed.

Focus is the essence of martial arts movement. Non-martial artists starting martial dance will find this, plus the hand and foot coordination, the most problematic part of the lesson. Focus is not natural, it is almost unique to Budo since no other sport demands it to such an extent, and compared with the martial arts it is only used sparingly in contemporary dance and ballet. It is the art of stopping an exactly executed technique dead at its completion point. Focus is the ability not only to make a technique look powerful and pin-point precise, but to arrest its trajectory in an instant so that the power that is generated can almost be seen to be catapulted out of the end of the hand or foot that has just performed the punch, strike, block or kick.

Nevertheless not all movements have a fast, hard focus; some of them have a softer focus, a more gentle and flowing nature, but no movements are weak or ambiguous — this would be a cardinal sin in martial dance. All movements have a definite beginning, trajectory and sharp completion point. Different types of movement — tension movements, fast, hard, staccato movements and soft, flowing movements are also highlighted.

When a technique needs a special focus and emphasis it is sometimes appropriate to **kiai** or shout. It does not matter what one shouts as long as it is an abstract sound. Kiai helps to liberate the spirit and dispel inhibitions. The shout may fall on a prearranged movement or be spontaneous.

AEROBICS

Martial dance can be performed to all types of music but in the lesson most of the music will be pop and rock. **Aerobics** involve some simple punching and kicking techniques which are performed to music; the primary aim of these is to build up fitness. A long record is chosen and a series of martial techniques are unravelled for its entire duration. Depending on the experience of the students, this non-stop aerobic workout can last from five to fifteen minutes, involving two or three changes of music.

SELF-DEFENCE

The lesson is designed to alternate the mental and physical aspects of martial dance, so recovery times are provided after stamina work by concentrating on technique. For example, after aerobics, which is fitness training, there follows self-defence which is technical and less demanding on the lungs.

In the **self-defence** section, all or some of the techniques that are about to be used in the actual martial dance routines are investigated with respect to their self-defence application. This involves a close examination of technique and practice of these attacks and counter-attacks with a partner. It involves learning vulnerable target areas and rehearsing controlled strikes, punches and kicks to these areas. It is also important to include the psychology of self-protection, the necessity for spirit and confidence in a life-threatening situation.

POWER TRAINING

Ideally the martial dancer should train on punch bags or striking pads. The techniques should be learned from the inside out, so gaining an empathy with them. None of the movements are pure dance movements, they are *martial* dance movements. Martial means warlike, and these movements must be performed from the soul of a warrior. As techniques they must have a cutting edge, a lethal potential. The emphasis in martial dance is on peace, but if all connection was lost with the martial roots it would become effete and devoid of integrity. Martial dance is peace-promoting not pacifist.

The martial dancer will perform with more conviction knowing he or she can use these techniques, knowing, that is, that he or she can back up the dance of power with real power. **Power** is generated and developed by constant practice on striking pads which can be held by students working in pairs. Sometimes the finer points of technique only cease to be theoretical and abstract when the student actually hits a target. Pad work can also be very good for fitness training.

ON THE SPOT ROUTINES

At this stage in the lesson we are ready to start actually dancing. The **spot routines** can be performed by many students in unison. They usually last about five seconds each and students should learn at least twenty or thirty — there is in fact no limit, so they can be alternated to a record. The usual number to use for one piece of music is four and each one is performed for four or five repetitions before smoothly slipping into the next one. The changeover can be prearranged or signalled by the teacher. An advanced student will be able to do ten or even twenty routines to one record if it is so desired.

Spot routines are a good test of memory, coordination, focus, balance, suppleness and rhythm. At first the student will have difficulty with the coordination, and then with the task of memorizing the sequence of movements well enough for them to become automatic. But with perseverence and concentration, these are no obstacles of any consequence.

FREE DANCE

Free dance is a more advanced form of martial dance than spot routines, although there is no sharp division between the two — in fact spot routines should be regarded as units that one can introduce into free dance. It is called free dance because the dancer is freed from the spatial limitations of on-the-spot dancing. In free dance, because of the stances, there is a much more ambitious utilization of floor space.

The student is now taught to link the stances together, covered in basics, to form sequences and cultivate the rhythmic body movements that further identify martial dance and differentiate it from traditional kata. Now everything is brought together — breathing, timing, tension poses, soft movements, hard movements, slow movements, fast movements, stances, spinning kicks, spot routines, multiples. Sequences involving some or all of these aspects are learned by constant repetition and filed away in the mind to enrich the kinetic vocabulary of the dancer. The advanced student is encouraged to practise improvisation by drawing on this reservoir of knowledge and invoking random units. The free dance sequences are taught one technique at a time, and when the whole sequence is learned it is practised without music to begin with. Before a whole sequence can be performed to music, some time must be spent practising how to move rhythmically while locked into a stance or while moving from one stance or pose to another.

Finally, the class ends with a visualization exercise in which the free dance sequence is practised not just for its physical benefits but for strengthening the psyche. This is dealt with in more detail in the next chapter.

ATTITUDE

The ideal student is rare in any field of human endeavour. But it is never just a matter of physical aptitude — the **mental attitude,** the frame of mind, is of equal if not greater importance. In the martial arts few people stay the course even to black belt, which is only the beginning, the point at which in martial arts terms the student reaches adulthood. Few people have the character to search for the heart of an art by peeling away the layers of meaning through relentless effort.

Mental maturity is the ability to perceive a worthwhile cause, to select a life-goal and to strive for perfection. It is because of the importance of the mind in training that the martial dance lesson includes reminders of the underlying principles of the art. Understanding a little of the philosophy of martial dance will help the student to maintain interest and enthusiasm. To understand *why* you train as well as how is of immense importance. Motivation is sustained by idealism.

7

VISUALIZATION

It is incumbent upon the teacher at the close of the lesson, before the final enactment of the free dance sequence to music, to engender in the student's mind a positive mental disposition — the mind-power of the warrior. It is necessary to the true spirit of martial dance that the student leaves the class feeling that both body and mind have been exercised and that the act of performing martial dance has helped in getting attuned to nature and in heightening awareness of reality, even if this is only in some cases to reaffirm and consolidate self-evident truths.

In this way the closing dances become, in the mind of the serious student, the physical correlation of a concept — the bodily expression of a mental construct. By a simple **visualization exercise** the warrior spirit is generated through the body. To understand this primal power it is necessary to construe life itself as a mode of combat in which the human spirit — the fighting spirit — is being continually tested with challenges of one kind or another. To survive and win this battle of existence one needs power in its various forms, especially the willpower, and it is this truth — that life itself is strife — that makes us all warriors, whether we know it or not. We have no choice but to fight. If this is the stark reality of our human condition, then everything that can help us generate the fighting spirit, the will to power, is of great use to us.

The teacher must remind his class of the classical martial arts perspective on reality. The dance itself now becomes an affirmation of the fact that one is a warrior, in fact a microcosm of one's own life, which one dances or lives out as a person who has awakened to his warrior identity, his martial self-image. The dancer must dance not as a weak person but as a being

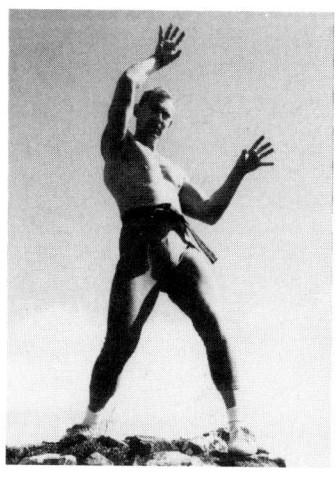

Human life and indeed all human history would be inconceivable without the element of struggle. Although it is unpleasant to think of society solely in terms of power — which can lead to violence — power is undeniably a determining factor in human fate. Of the various kinds of power, virtue is the highest; and a society in which struggle is limited to competition in developing and manifesting virtue would no doubt be optimum. Unfortunately in actuality, struggle takes place on all levels from low personal interest to lofty ideals. And, in all these combats, it is important to strive to win. Even in cases of defeat, however, it is possible to learn much that must be used for the sake of victory in coming struggles.

Mas Oyama
(The Kyokushin Way)

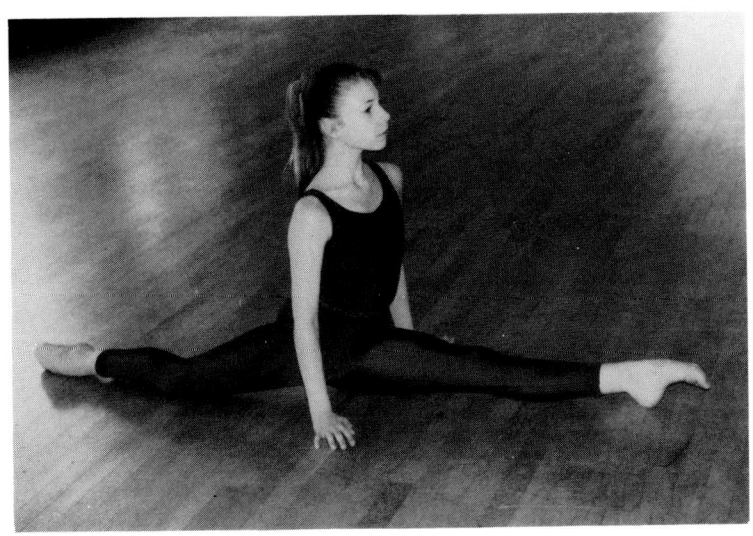

of power and self-confidence — the dancer must dance as he would like to live. In the dance you are the master of your own destiny; you control your body and your balance, and you decide which stance you adopt and how long you hold it. At this time students never dance in unison for they express their own individuality and decide when, where, and how to move. For a while these visualization dances are set patterns prescribed by the teacher but eventually students will reach a degree of proficiency that will enable them to improvise.

The first move of such a dance is always the same. The dancer stands with the feet together and the eyes closed, the hands outstretched with the palms facing upwards level with the waist. The hands then describe a circle and meet at the top above eye level with the palms facing down. This circle symbolizes the sun, and immortality. The sun is the life-giver, sustaining all life on the planet. The teacher then asks his students to visualize their warrior spirit as a glowing energy field concentrated just below the navel but emanating its power outwards through the body. When this has been judged by each individual to have been achieved, he or she may continue their power dance. Just as in Ram Muay the Thai Boxer believes he can improve his chances of victory by visualizing himself beforehand, destroying his opponent, so the martial dancer believes that when the lesson is over the ritual dance will have activated psycho-physical forces that will enhance the individual's chances of success in everyday life.

The visualization dance is usually performed to instrumental music to avoid distracting lyrics, and it is repeated until the end of the music, each time recommencing with the first movement and the attendant mental imagery.

The power centre just below the navel is traditional in the martial arts and is called 'T'an Tien' — a Taoist term which refers to the sleeping energies in people. As one does chi-building exercises such as tai-chi, energy gradually develops and is stored in this area. This however is not the only reason for choosing such a locality. It is logical that the life force should be visualized as existing in close proximity to the organs of procreation. It also feels right because in a relaxed standing position one's centre of gravity is located approximately at the navel.

8

SACRED DANCE

Dance has at many times in the past been a magical ritual, a religious ceremony or a sacrament. The nearest we have to it today outside the martial arts are ballet and contemporary dance, which are often used to express, on a personalized level, the concepts of a particular choreographer. These cannot compare, in terms of emotive power, with the deep rooted religious beliefs that are shared by a whole tribe or civilization and endowed with the weight of tradition. Dance is truly sacred when it expresses the soul of a nation or the collective religious aspirations of a group. Budo is, for those who can discern its deeper levels, a religion, a way of life, and it is the function of martial dance to express the soul of its philosophy.

Pre-scientific peoples frequently engaged in ritualistic dancing. When they needed sun or rain they summoned the tribe and danced a sun dance or a rain dance, and for them the act of dancing had magical power. When they wanted to hunt and catch a bear they would rehearse the hunt in a bear dance. In many primitive societies as a person passed from childhood to youth and from youth to manhood, so the number of dances increased and the number of these dances was the measure of social importance. Dance for these people was a way of generating psychic energy. A tribe about to go to war would work itself up into a frenzy of aggression by performing a war dance. There were also fertility dances to raise sexual energy and to ensure the fertility of the land.

SACRED DANCE OF THE NORTH AMERICAN INDIAN

The **North American Indian** is well-known for his warrior prowess, but he was also a great nature lover. The dances of

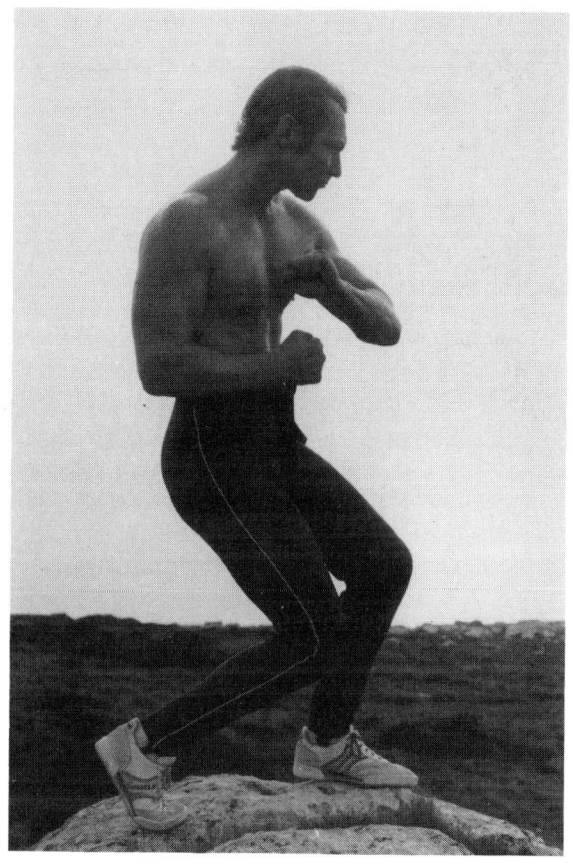

If music is related to the movements of the hands and feet and entire body, it results in something like dance. It is this dance element that reflects in karate.

Mas Oyama
(This is Karate)

the Indians were a way of expressing their deep spirituality, giving them a profound relationship, an empathy, with their beautiful surroundings.

Some Plains tribes performed the **Sun Dance** every summer and sometimes self-mutilation was practised. The purpose of the ritual was to renew communion with the earth, wind, sun and the spirits, so that the tribe might have health and fertility and the buffalo might never fail. Every movement was a prayer understood by all, and many of the dancers played eagle-bone whistles, which represented the 'Thunderbird' and were used to summon rain. The eagle was the patron of war and was thus invoked in spirit by the ritual. The element of self-torture, involving being suspended by thongs through the chest, was a sacrifice of what was most precious to them — their own flesh and blood. It was meant to convince the powers of their earnestness in seeking supernatural help.

One of the most poignant examples of dance taking on an almost unique profundity is the **Ghost Dance**. This tragic dance was also accompanied by apocalyptic warrior songs. Towards the end of the nineteenth century, traditional lifestyles began to fade for the Indians. Many were moved off their homelands by settlers from the Old World, and in their despair they waited for some miracle to rescue them from misery. Then the rumour grew and spread like wildfire — the Great Spirit had taken pity on his Indian children, and he would make a new world. A great flood would come and the old earth would roll itself up like a carpet revealing the fresh new earth beneath. A great medicine man had been annointed for the mission in the south. All the Indians had to do to bring this new world about was to dance the ghost dance, which the prophet would teach them.

They would have to dance each month for four days wearing a feather so that the Great Spirit could tell them at a glance. If they did this, all would come to pass as foretold within two years. Warriors travelled to meet the prophet and learn the dance and songs. In their high emotional states they easily succumbed to visions and trances. Men and women were given ghost dance shirts that were bullet proof in case anyone attempted to interfere by attacking the dancers. They were taught how to dance in a circle, men and women holding hands, facing always towards the centre. They had only their own voices to accompany them, because this was a dance without drums or any other instruments. In this way they danced hour after hour without food or water until they dropped in a dead faint. Sometimes a dancer broke out of the circle, his arms outstretched towards the horizon, his eyes closed, trembling, seeing with his inward eye the vision of the promised land, his mind ablaze with the sad and noble hopes of his doomed brothers and sisters.

As taught by the prophet, the new religion was entirely peaceful. He did not teach the destruction of the newcomers; he taught only that they would go away. The new world could not be brought about by bloodshed. Even among the warlike tribes no violence was contemplated. Why expose oneself to slaughter and suffering, said the leaders, when the new world will come by itself?

The American Indian lived in a beautiful country full of space, bright light, eagles and dramatic scenery. He was a God-intoxicated being. He saw God not as a transcendent being but as suffusing the universe, and he worshipped God *through* His creation. It was because the Indians' way of life was suffused with nature worship that their sacred dances were so profound and expressive. Through dance they gained communion with the universe. Today we must relearn this.

THE SACRED DANCE OF SUFISM

The time-honoured liaison between religion, dance, and ecstatic experience is further embodied in Sufism — a variant of Islam. Sufism proposes to reach God through trance states induced by dancing. The Sufi wants an immediate ecstatic experience of oneness with God, and the means to accomplish this is a once-secret rite of twirling dance movements — hence the term 'whirling dervish'.

It is said that to master this twirling motion over a thousand hours of training are required; devotees also chant while they dance and eventually they enter a trance state. This esoteric ecstasy cult demonstrates the power of dance and music to affect the mind, especially if they are coupled with a profound and emotive idea. Dance can energize a belief with feeling and help weld it into the psyche.

THE WILL TO POWER

Martial dance like any other dance can be a fun recreation, an aerobic exercise, or an art-form, but its quintessence is ritualism and it celebrates the maxim of the 'will to power'. By dancing, one not only wills oneself into a powerful and positive state of mind that carries over into everyday life, one is also commemorating the fact that we need power in all its different forms to live and to succeed in life. The warrior way is the way of power.

With visualization techniques and by identifying with nature, the practitioner of martial dance becomes one with the universe. By visualizing oneself as a forcefield blending with other forcefields, flowing with nature like a river, one feels the life force. This life force has many aspects and one of its most important is the procreative force or the sex drive.

THE PROCREATIVE FORCE

The thrusting hip movements of martial dance are its most unorthodox and seemingly irreverent quality. Whereas dance is usually erotic, whether it is trying to be or not, traditional kata is relatively cold and clinical. In the transition from kata to dance, erotic sensuality begins to emerge. This is unavoidable because music and the body itself are intrinsically sensual. The pelvic pushes are essential for hooking onto the beat on the occasions when the tempo of the music demands it and keeping the stances from becoming too static.

Apart from this pragmatic justification, such rhythmic hip movement is unashamedly symbolic of the procreative force. Budo has a tradition of Eastern philosophy and metaphysics, and in its heritage can be found the explicit eroticism of Japanese Shinto and Hindu Tantrism. Dance and sexuality have always been inseparable soulmates. The procreative force is sacred, as the aforementioned religions affirmed, because the power that creates new life is the greatest power of all. In every dance the martial dancer automatically celebrates the power that brought him or her into the world.

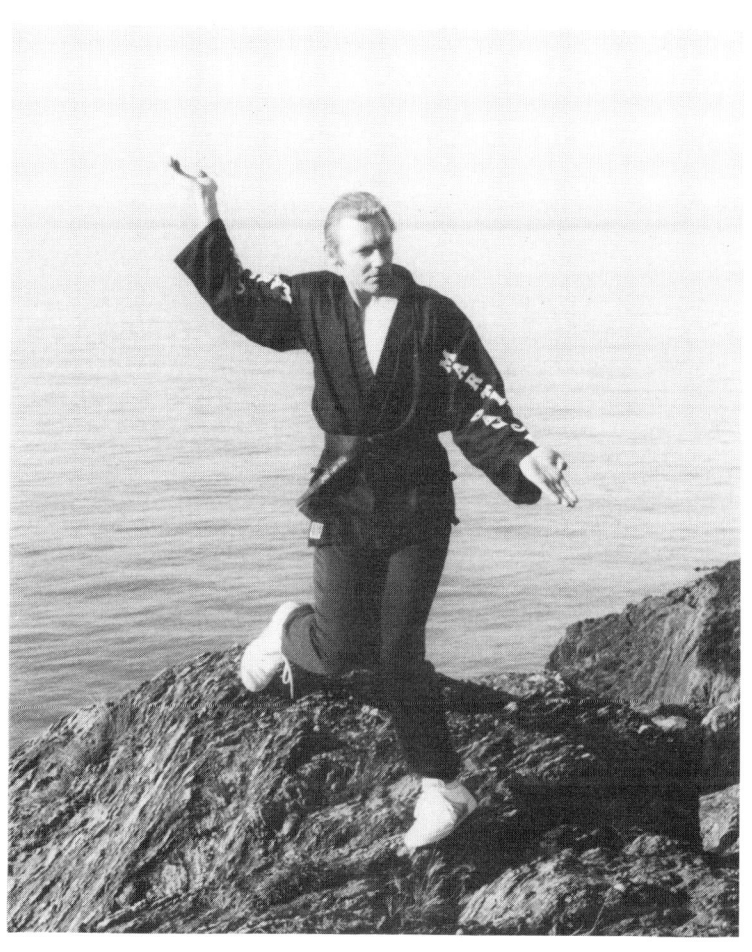

SPONTANEOUS DANCE

The advanced martial dancer arrives at the point where he can perform a spontaneous or creative dance in which he improvises from the vast storehouse of martial movements that derive from years of training. He dances from his soul and his unconscious. In this way he expresses his being at that particular point in time rather than regurgitating a pre-set routine, which could be seen from one point of view as something lifeless: something born of and in bondage to the past, needing to be reanimated and therefore lacking spontaneity.

Zen Buddhism emphasizes the importance of living in the here and now, and this idea of creative dance perfectly embodies the concept of spontaneity, of recreating oneself in the fresh intensity of the now. In this way dance is born that vanishes, for all time, in the very process of creation.

HARMONY OF BODY AND MIND

We are all fortunate to be alive and to be the proud owners of our bodies, which are marvellously complex machines, and it is a moral duty to maintain them. The body is the energizing centre of man's spirituality, and the mind is the intellectual powerhouse behind all social progress and scientific evolution.

Man is a duality of mind and body, and martial dance reflects this by being both physical and mental. Its movements are physical in outward appearance but are also expressions of mental states and precepts. Behind them the dancer's mind releases ideas that permeate the dance. Martial dance is a form of philosophical meditation and before each dance a treasured belief should be selected for cogitation and the dance performed with this in mind so that it becomes a celebration of one's faith.

The reason for martial dance itself is that there must be a correlation between mind and body. The body's movements should reflect the motions of the mind and in this way mind and body are unified. Martial dance is, therefore, spiritually holistic. Furthermore, in dance the soul, or one's psychic centre of passion and feeling, is activated and brought into play to energize and fortify the mind. The soul is spirit; without spirit you cannot dance or fight well.

9

MARTIAL DANCE — A CONTRADICTION?

It is natural that some people might look askance at the paradox of a non-violent martial art. They ask, no doubt, whether a tradition of fighting skills should be interpreted in this way. Underlying such suspicions there is often a prejudice against serious forms of dance such as ballet because they are deemed weak or effeminate.

As a counter-argument to this, it can be said that martial dance, though peace-promoting, is not pacifist but recognizes the importance of self-defence and retains this traditional element within itself. Non-violence in connection with martial dance does not therefore mean that violence is ruled out as a last resort, but it does mean that it is de-emphasized in comparison with most martial arts. Added to this, if this art is non-aggressive, it is only so in a certain sense of the term. There are different modes of expressing aggression. If by aggression we mean a no-nonsense tenacity in pursuance of some task or ambition, or the warrior-spirit, then martial dance does certainly express it.

Violence is on the increase in the streets discos, and in the clubland jungle, and the martial arts world has not, on the whole, helped matters very much. In most training halls and dojos the spiritual aspects of the martial arts are seldom mentioned and the emphasis is on competition, fighting, and learning often deadly techniques. In martial arts movies, fighting is glamourized and made into a gymnastic melodrama. Films that try and investigate the deeper side of the arts like *The Silent Flute* are few and far between.

Added to this, the continual emphasis on aggression in combat is a subtle influence and engenders in some students, even if it is subconscious, a desire to put theory into practice and see how well the techniques work.

To appreciate the significance of martial dance as a non-competitive and potentially civilizing force in society, it is important to remember the bellicosity of the present social climate. We in the twentieth century have inherited the legacy of thousands of years of bloodletting and violent conquest. Men, as individuals and as nations, have usually settled their differences with the sword rather than with reason.

Many people believe that war is sometimes necessary — the glory of war and the warrior ideal are not total misconceptions; they are just overplayed and oversimplified. Behind all the violence we find the spectre of the male principle. Men, not women, are mostly responsible for violence from wars to soccer hooliganism, rape, robbery, and mugging. The warrior hero is in our cultural bloodstream, but in martial dance there is an attempt to modify the machismo to suit new needs.

THE ARCHETYPAL WARRIOR HERO

Our society is heavily imbued with the drama of combat. Almost every film on our TV or cinema screens depicts at some point the spectacle of a villain's defeat at the noble hands of a hero who has all the requisite hallmarks of the archetype: good looks, a strong body, and matchless fighting skills, together with the reckless courage to use them at any opportunity which presents itself. We all love a hero but have things gone too far? Have we allowed ourselves to be seduced by the drama of violence for its own sake?

The martial folk heros have multiplied in our mass media world to take on a profusion of bizarre forms from the fantasy cartoon to the surrealistic realms of science fiction. From this medley of combative superbeings have emerged such characters as Superman, Tarzan, Rocky, and countless others, all vicariously satisfying our deep urge to experience the danger and glory of man to man combat.

These superheroes are nearly always male, which rules out half the human species from this extravaganza of narcissism. They illustrate the self-projection of man into the realm of fiction which he uses like a magic mirror to gaze upon his own idealized self-image. They abound in endless permutations from the sublime to the ridiculous. Some of them, unique to the modern world, use science to extend their powers. The archetype then takes on the protean forms of the hi-tech megaheroes with bionic implants or with back up from futuristic motorbikes, cars, or helicopters. They have become part of our TV folk culture and are continually upstaged by ever more fantastic creations.

Within the syndrome of the tough-guy hero there is often the undertone of eroticism, as with the rescue of maidens in distress. Our culture reinforces a man's natural tendency to impress women with his physical strength and martial abilities — his inborn mating dance. In most action movies women are portrayed as helpless victims of their supposed physical inferiority; they are totally dependent on men in any situation that hinges on personal initiative or martial abilities. It is no wonder that hitherto women have been largely excluded from the cult of the warrior hero. This is why in Martial Dance the aforementioned archetype must be feminized — this does not mean, of course, that it must be made weak or effeminate, but that its hard, aggressive, and destructive side must be counter-balanced with the creative and peace-promoting aspects of the whole.

It is against this backdrop of male violence that the female principle has so much to contribute. It has been repressed for too long and it is now beginning to re-establish itself in an equal and harmonious relationship with its opposite.

ANTI-VIOLENCE AND THE FEMALE PRINCIPLE

The clarion call of feminism, which has sounded its criticisms, insights, and convictions over the last few decades, may, like any other movement, have its share of misconceptions, but it has changed the way we view women and their role in the future.

It may or may not be a myth that women are the more peace-loving sex, but it is certainly true the pressures on them to be violent and to live up to some ideal of Martial heroism are virtually non-existent. They are not expected to mimic a bar-brawling John Wayne or the xenophobic antics of a flag-waving

Rambo. For this reason the female principle can be understood as less orientated to violence, and more likely to aid the redefinition of the warrior ideal, through the agency of martial dance.

10

YIN/YANG HARMONY —
THE EASTERN CONNECTION

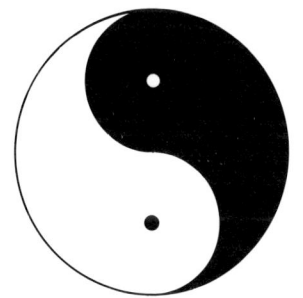

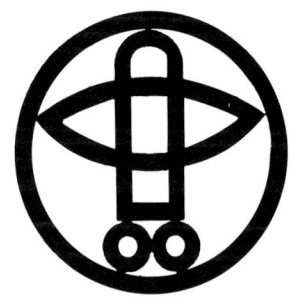

1 *Yin/Yang Symbol*   **2** *Life Force Logo*

TAOISM

Martial dance can help to restore the balance of yin and yang within each of us. The question of the balance of opposites is dealt with in some depth in the Taoist religion, which has had a formative influence on the martial arts.

The emblem on the top left is the yin/yang symbol, which represents the female and male forces respectively. We see that a black spot resides in the white shape and a white spot in the black. This illustrates the fact that each gender has within itself the seed of its opposite.

Taoism maintains that the dynamism of the cosmos is the result of the interplay between opposites, namely the yin and yang — elemental gender forces. We needn't take this mytho-poetic idea as absolutely literal, but the concept behind it is true. Yin and yang symbolize the tension of opposites, the polarization of life and ultimately a transcendence of opposites to a unity beyond.

Opposite the yin/yang symbol is the emblem of martial dance

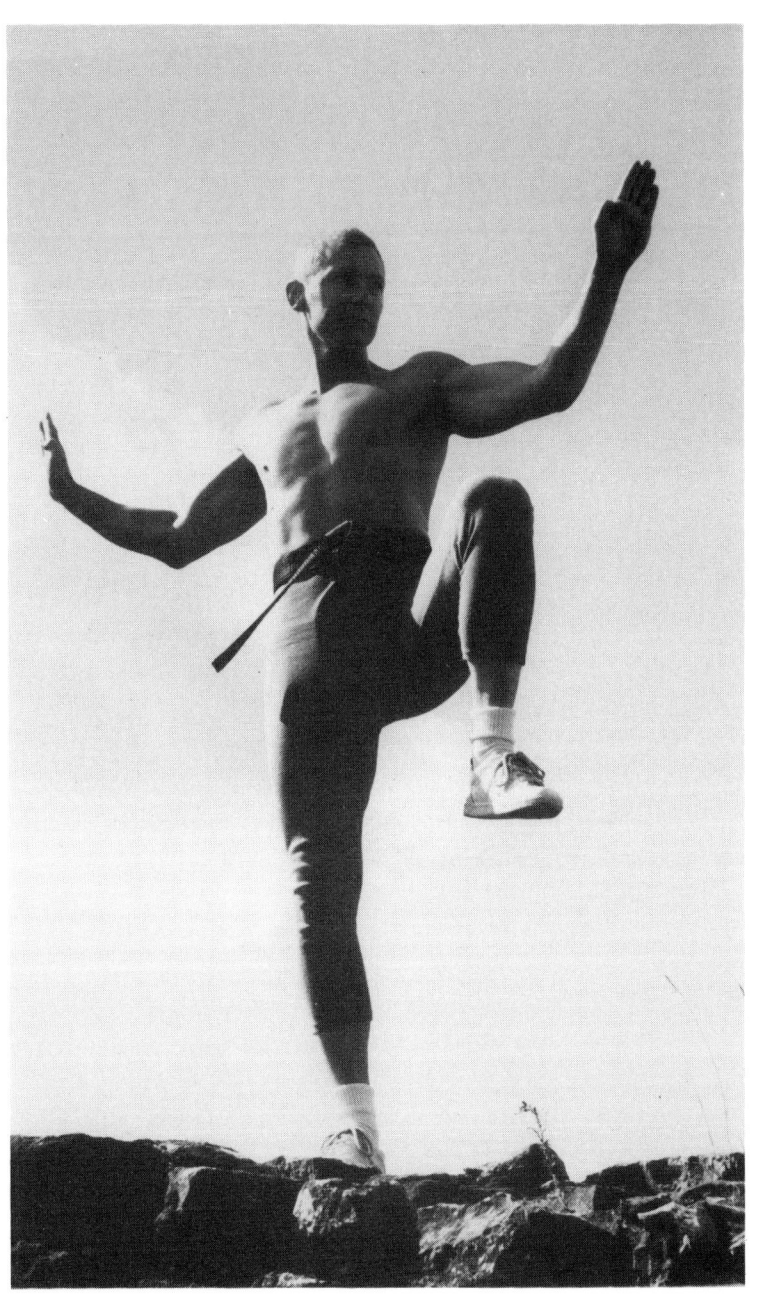

— the life force logo. It manifests the male and female principles in harmony and celebrates not only the ultimate oneness of the universe but the procreative energy of nature. Around this energy is the circle, symbolizing the sun which sustains all life on our planet.

The religions of the East, through which the martial arts have developed, all have a dimension that affirms the erotic energy of nature. Even Zen Buddhism endorses a positive attitude to the life force. Taisen Deshimaru, a Zen master born of a Samurai family, explained in *The Zen Way To The Martial Arts:* 'Cosmic energy is concentrated in the lower abdomen and especially in the genital organs . . . When procreation occurs, sexual energy is the vehicle whereby the force (ki) of universal life becomes manifest in the world of phenomena'.

We must remember that in our society the sex drive is often trivialized by being viewed at one extreme as an object of mirth and at the other as an obscenity. Its true purpose is often overlooked so we should remind ourselves from time to time that it is the means which nature has chosen for its lifeforms to perpetuate themselves. Sexual love is the manifest expression of nature's passion for continued and renewed existence.

Taisen Deshimura wrote of the recognition of this deeper meaning of the lifeforce.

It is important that modern education should restore an authentic, natural meaning to sexuality in our society. When it is understood as the energy from the life of the universe, sexuality adds a new quality to the relations between humans, brings love and human life to their highest dimension and brings true happiness.

SHINTO

Karate originated in Okinawa and Japan, and of the three contributory sources to the religious values of Japan — Buddhism, Confucianism, and Shinto — only the latter is indigenous to the country. Shinto means 'Way of the gods'. The sun was perceived as feminine, as a goddess, and held a central place in Shinto belief. Shinto is a nature religion and is often blatantly erotic. The nature spirits concerned with sexuality and love belonged to the land and its fertility.

In Shinto, sex has a transpersonal significance which is foreign to Western culture — in other words sex is seen as having a wider dimension beyond the mere personal relationship. The spirits personify the male and female principles in nature and were once represented in thousands of images and effigies at the roadsides and among the rice fields of peasant Japan. Male and female emblems of sexual energy usually couple in some way so as to represent the life force in action. Shinto shrines are often decorated with large sculptures of male and female sexual organs. There are even major temples in Japan which are entirely dedicated to the power of procreation.

DANCING THE LIFE FORCE

The martial dancer should exude an aura of power — it is the dance of power — but this is based on a broad interpretation, that is, a concept of power that allows the dancer to grow as a personality by exploring its dimensions. The life force is certainly one of the important aspects of personality, and this wonderful procreative ability derives from the union of opposites — male and female — brought together by the impulse of erotic love. But it is also the basic energy of life — the joy of life.

It is a fact that the art of dance is not just about technique or mechanical performance of the movements, for if the motion lacks the lifeforce — the very joy of being alive — they will be flat and dull. The energy of life has to animate a dancer's body and a good dancer is at his or her best when exhibiting the natural sexuality and sensuality of the human form in movement.

THE FIVE POWERS

Martial dance symbolizes five powers of the body — or, to be more precise, the mind/body duality. Of course, these powers cannot all be literally expressed through dance, but as a collective concept they underlie and lend structure to its deeper meaning. These are as follows:

1. Muscle Power.
2. Mind Power.

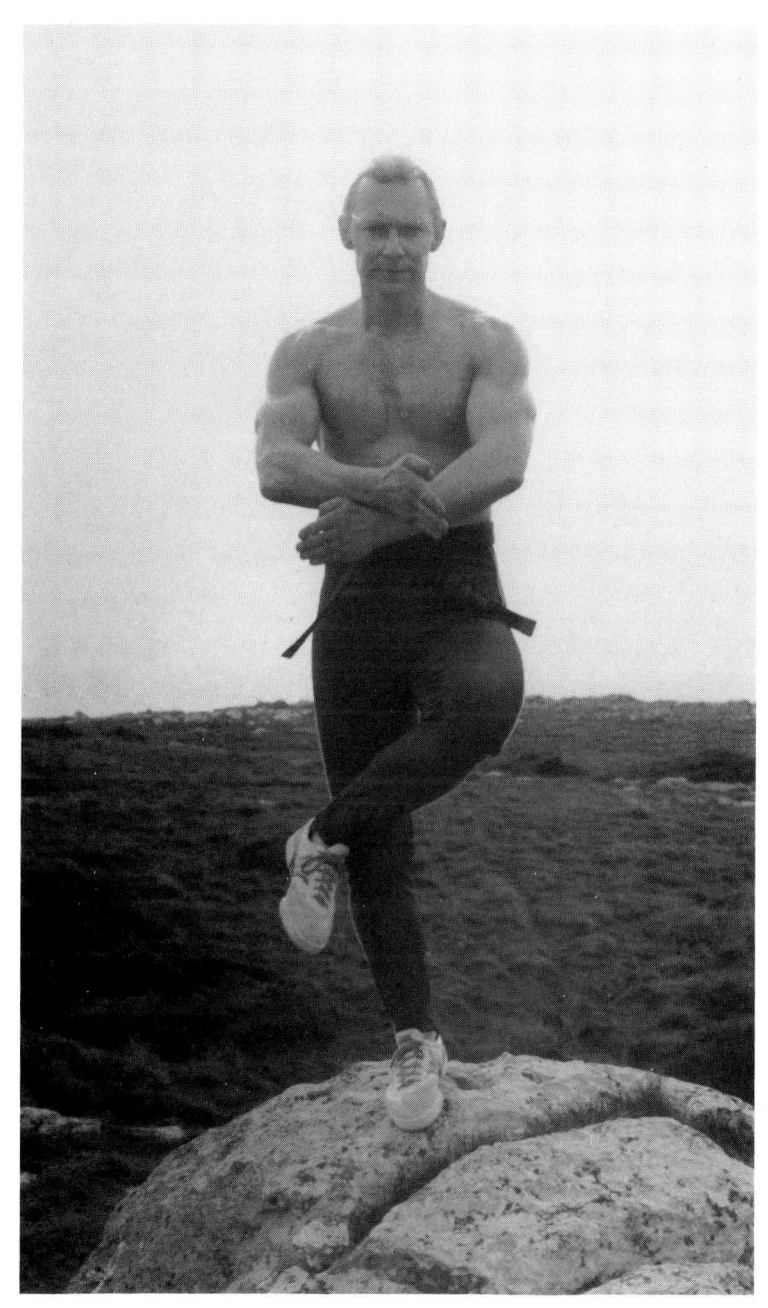

3. Willpower.
4. The Life Force.
5. Psychic Power.

The power of the muscles is the external power of the body which involves fitness and strength — the abilities one needs for good dance technique. The power of the mind is the reason and intuition that gives rise to philosophy, art, and science. This power filters our emotions and helps us to impose objective standards on our moral sentiments. The power of the will sustains us through adversity and fuels our efforts to realize our ambitions and aspirations, whereas the power of the life force is love of life, the instinct of self-preservation and the desire and ability to procreate.

Finally there is psychic power. Commonplace in the martial arts, and in bodybuilding, is the belief in 'mind over matter'. This concept is the first and most objective rung of the ladder of the hidden potential of mankind. This dimension of the human psyche is still largely uncharted and much remains to be investigated by many more years of scientific research. But mind over matter is the commonsense belief in positive thinking — the conviction that the mental disposition has the power to affect matter and the outcome of events.

Supernormal powers have been a constant theme running through the martial arts, where legend has merged with history. Where one draws the line to separate the two is a matter of personal choice. The Ninja, for example, were credited with the power to walk on water and render themselves invisible — which had at least a basis of fact. Certainly some martial artists can perform almost superhuman stunts like slicing through stones and bottles with their bare hands.

Many of the legends and reports that circulate in martial arts folklore are no doubt spurious, but there is nevertheless enough evidence of these powers to justify an open mind and further investigation. There have been many trustworthy eye witness accounts of experts and Grand Masters who have demonstrated powers that transcend the merely physical and border on the supernatural.

From ki, or internal power, to telepathy, invulnerability, clairvoyance, and telekinesis, the spectrum of psychic powers cannot be ignored. The powers of human potential must be reflected in the philosophy of martial dance and are projected symbolically through the dancer's body.

CONCLUSION

There is something exciting about living on the threshold of a new millennium. 2000 AD may be just a number, but it has a certain emotive ring to it which cannot be denied.

History is the manifestation of forces. Sometimes seemingly humble forces can contribute to changing a whole social climate. Aerobics, for example, has changed the lives and attitudes of millions of people — it has contributed to a new level of body consciousness.

Respect for one's body, health and fitness, is closely allied to respect for the sanctity of life, and from this one noble sentiment everything of value in human society emanates. Martial dance sets out to establish body awareness as a sacrament. This is part of the antidote, not only to runaway levels of drug and alchocol abuse and the escalation of wanton violence, but to the widespread spiritual bankruptcy of our times.

PART TWO
MARTIAL DANCE ROUTINES

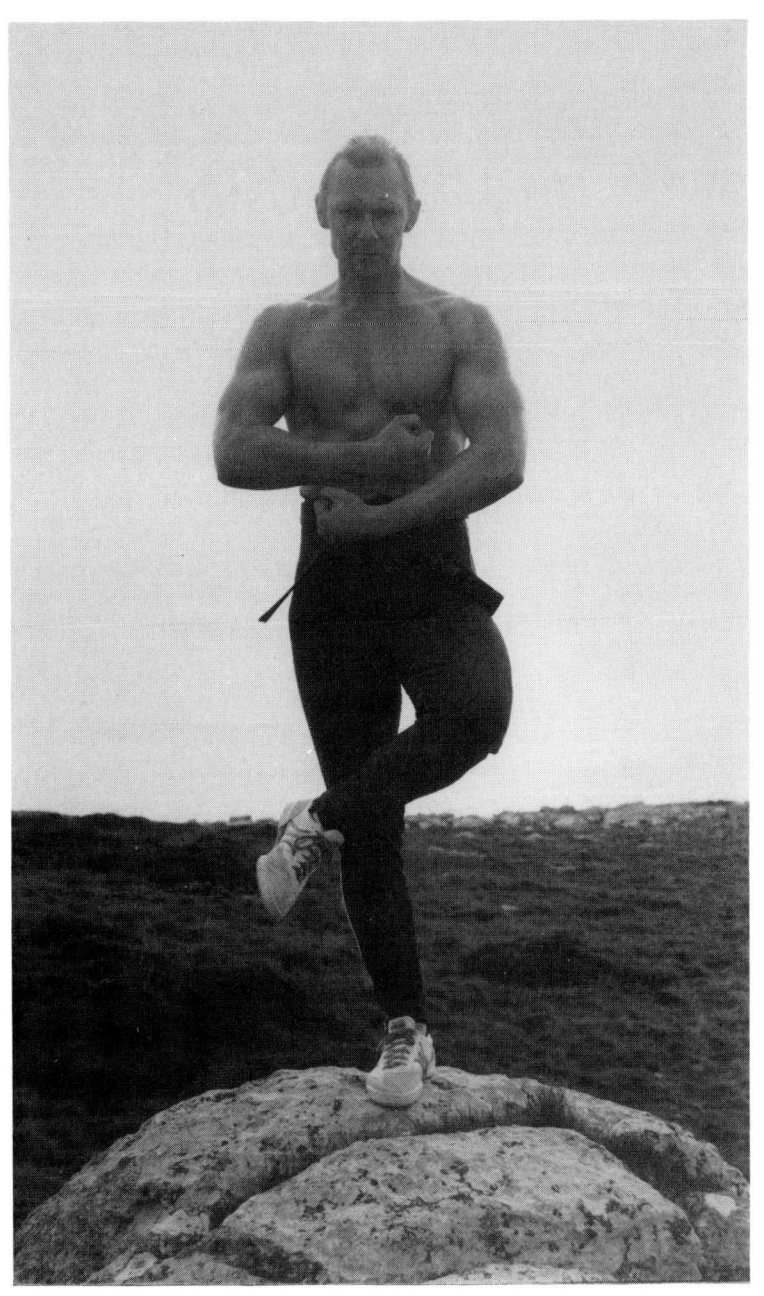

1

WARM-UPS AND STRETCHING

The exercises illustrated here are only a small selection from a wide range of possibilities. Stretching is helpful for high kicking as well as being beneficial to the health of the muscles.

Stretches should be done slowly and you should never bounce in a stretch. Rather, position yourself as specified and stretch the muscle until you feel a slight tension. Hold the position for about five to ten seconds and gently release. This allows the muscle to become accustomed to the position and to relax into it with a minimum of stress.

It is always a good thing not only to stretch before your main exercise programme but also after as part of your warm-down.

Wrist Exercise

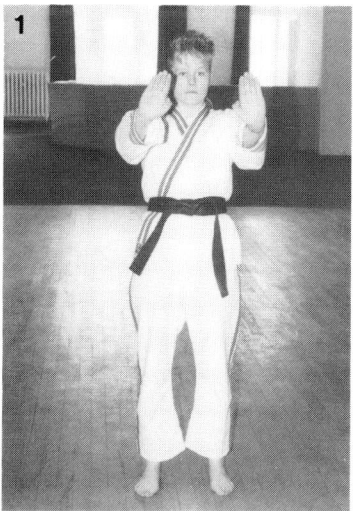

1 Hold your hands out with the palms facing outwards.

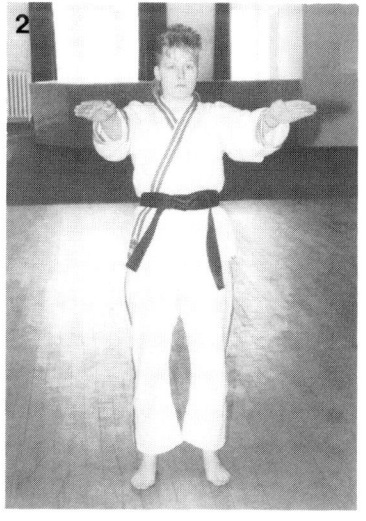

2 3 Turn in a circular motion.

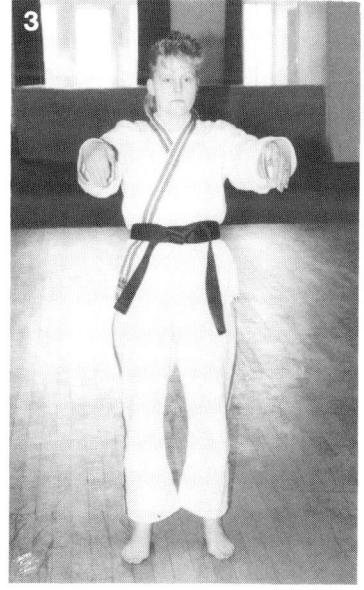

4 End the turn with palms facing inwards.

Neck Exercise

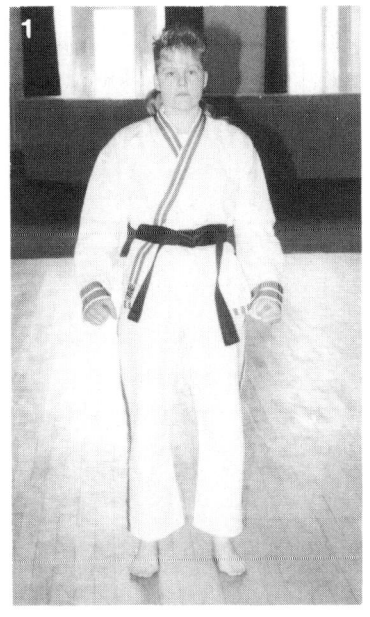

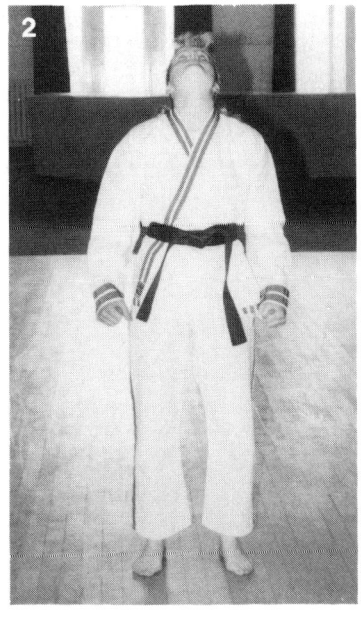

1 *Ready position.*

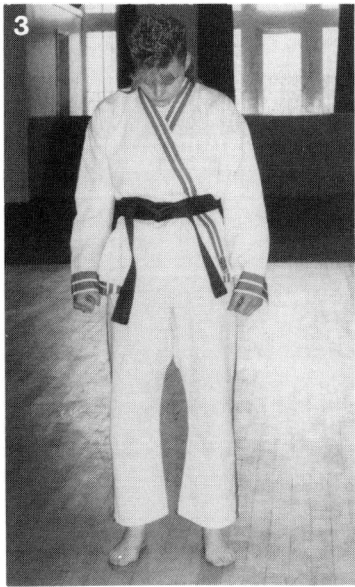

2 *Put your head back.*

3 *Put your head down.*

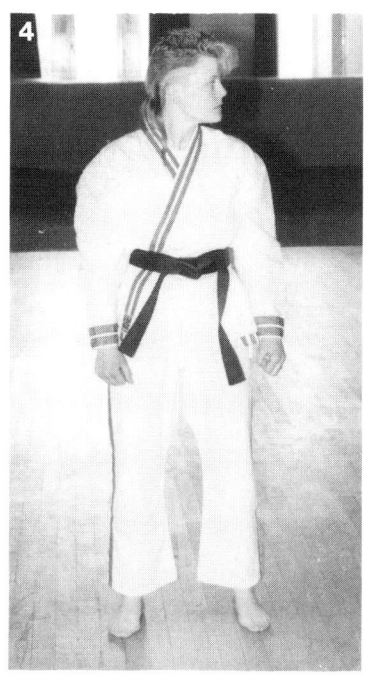

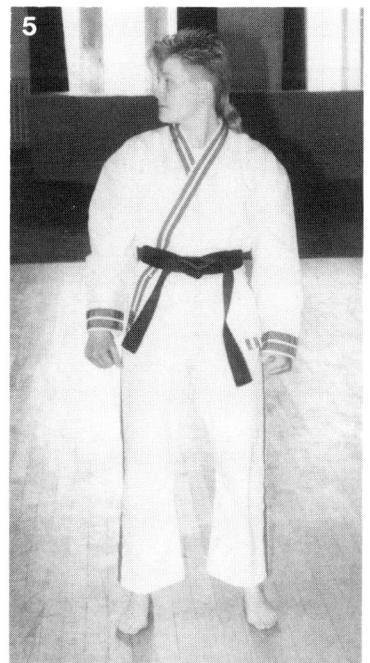

4 *Turn to the left.*

5 *Turn to the right.*

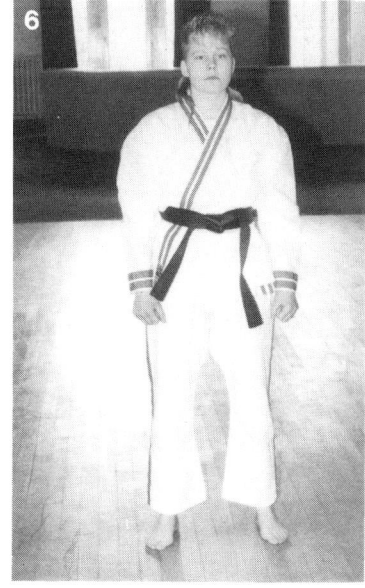

6 *Ready position — repeat the exercise.*

Side Bends.

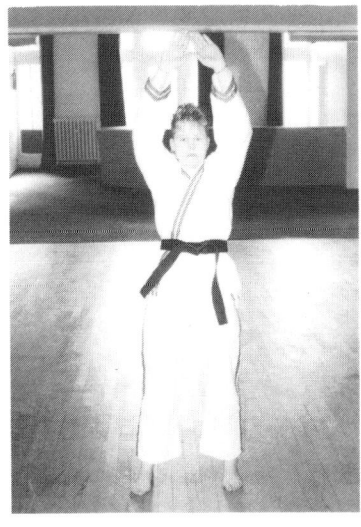

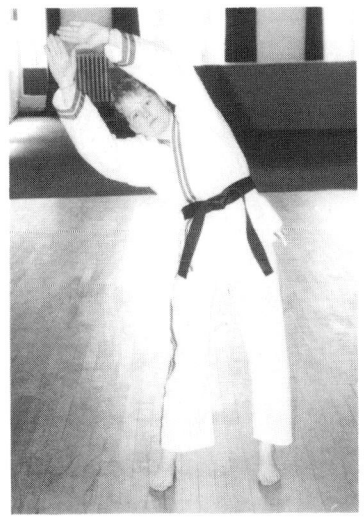

1 *Raise your hands above your head.*

2 *Bend to the right.*

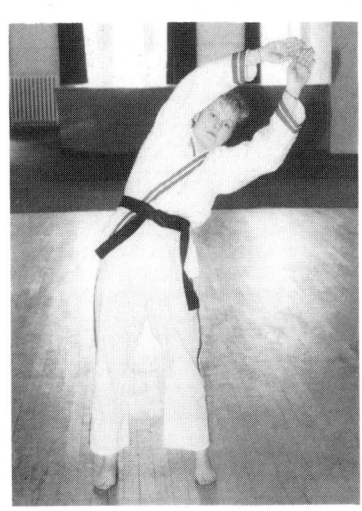

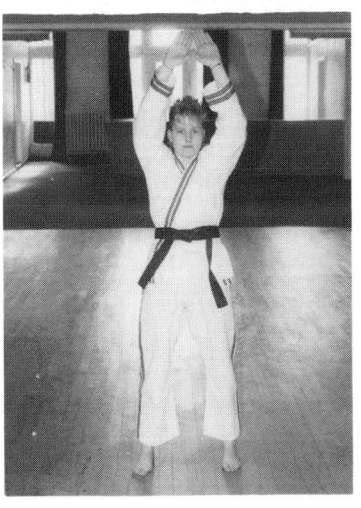

3 *Bend to the left.*

4 *Return to the starting position and repeat.*

Knee Pushdowns

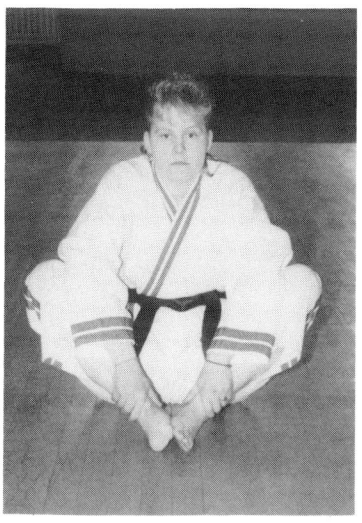

1 *Sit with your feet pulled up and place your elbows on your knees.*

2 *Push down your knees with your elbows.*

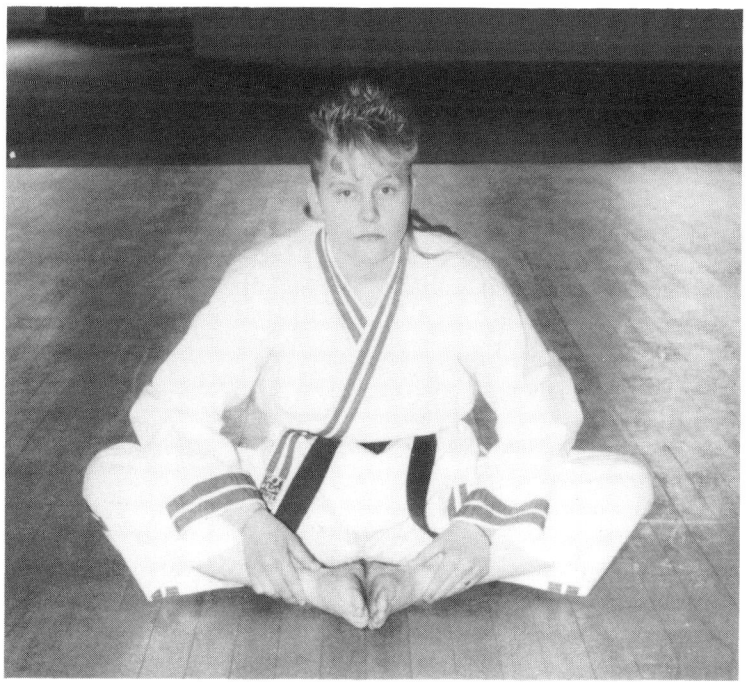

Leg Stretch I

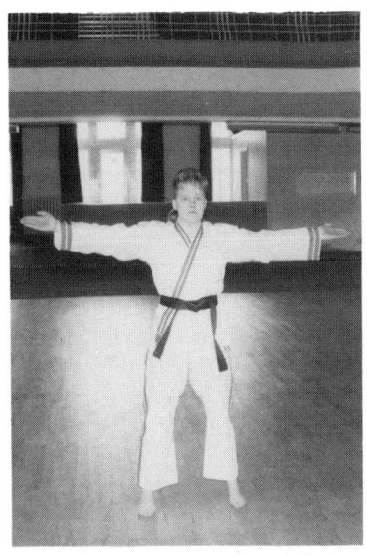 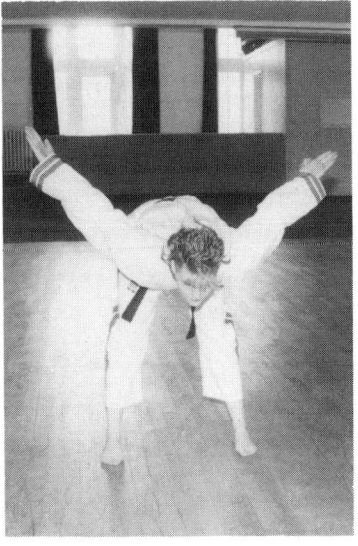

1 *Hold your hands out with your palms facing up.*

2 *Bend down slowly, turning your palms and keeping your legs straight.*

Leg Stretch II

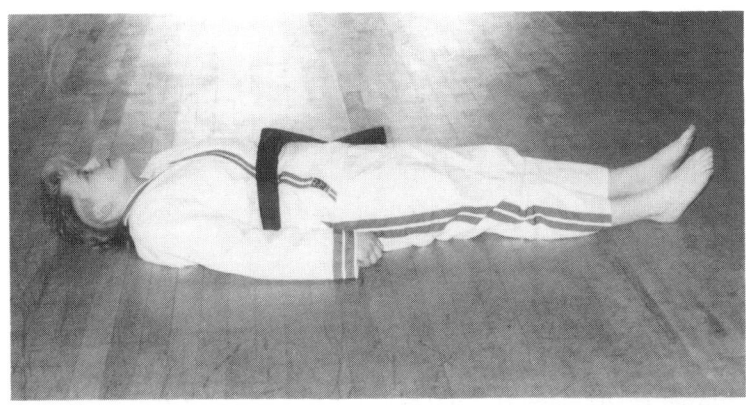

1 *Lie on your back.*

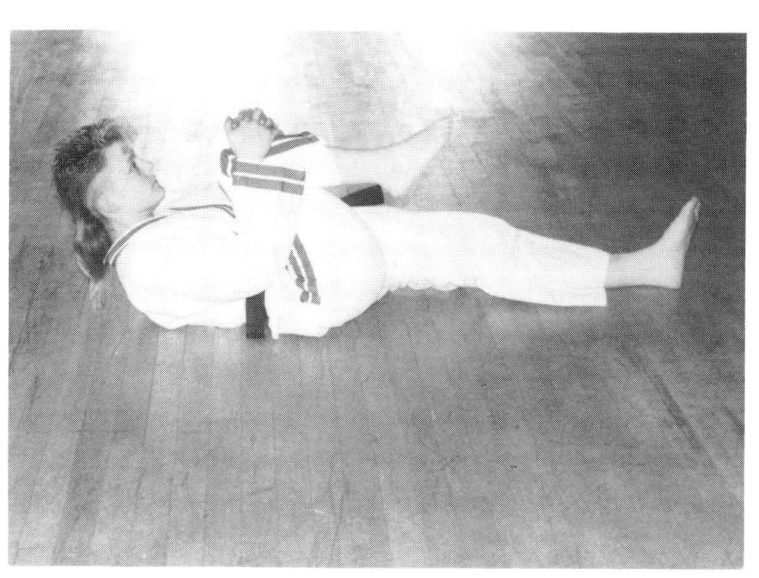

2 *Pull your right knee up.*

3 Straighten the leg and pull it towards you until you feel the stretch.

4 *Point and flex your foot. Then return to the starting position and repeat the exercise with your left leg.*

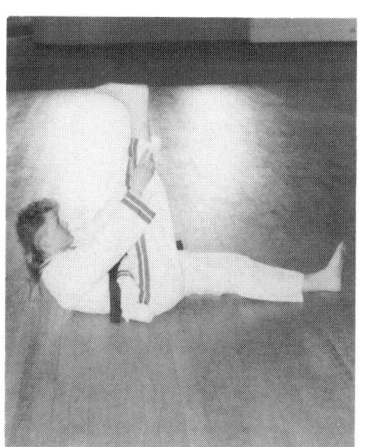

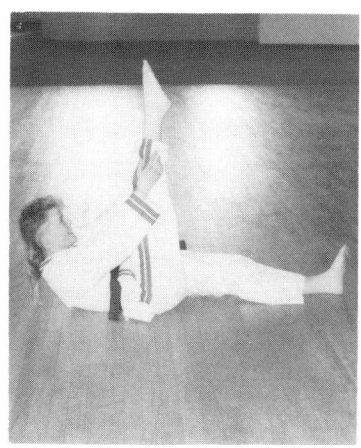

Leg Stretch III

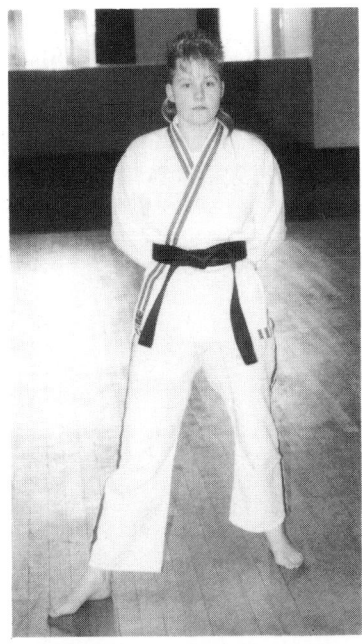

1 *Stand with your hands behind your back and your feet at right angles. Your right leg is in front of your left.*

2 *Bend down towards your leading leg which must remain straight at all times. Change your stance so that your left leg is in front and repeat the exercise for your left leg.*

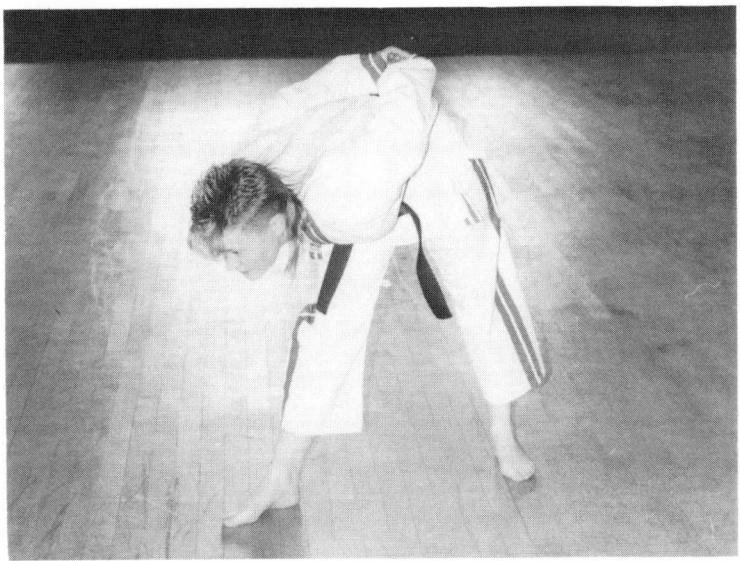

Leg Stretch IV

1 *Sit with your right leg tucked up and your left leg extended.*

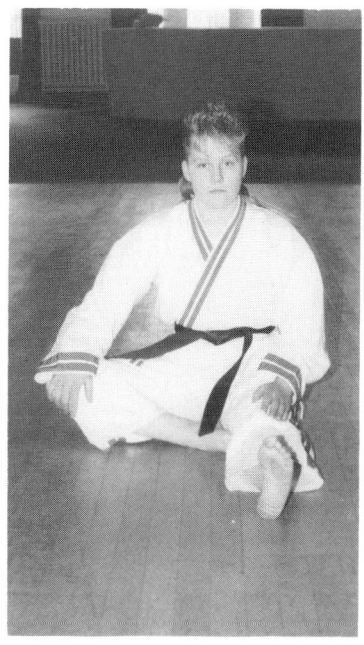

2 *Bend forward keeping your left leg flat on the floor and pushing your forehead towards your knee.*

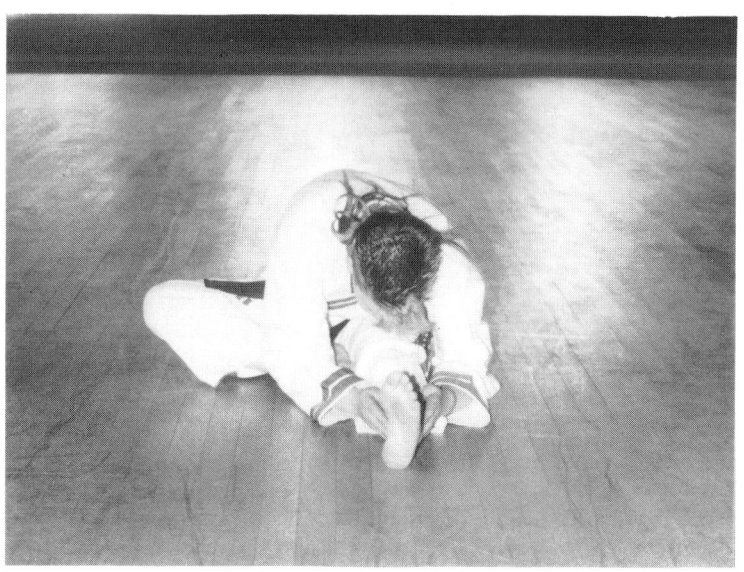

Splits I

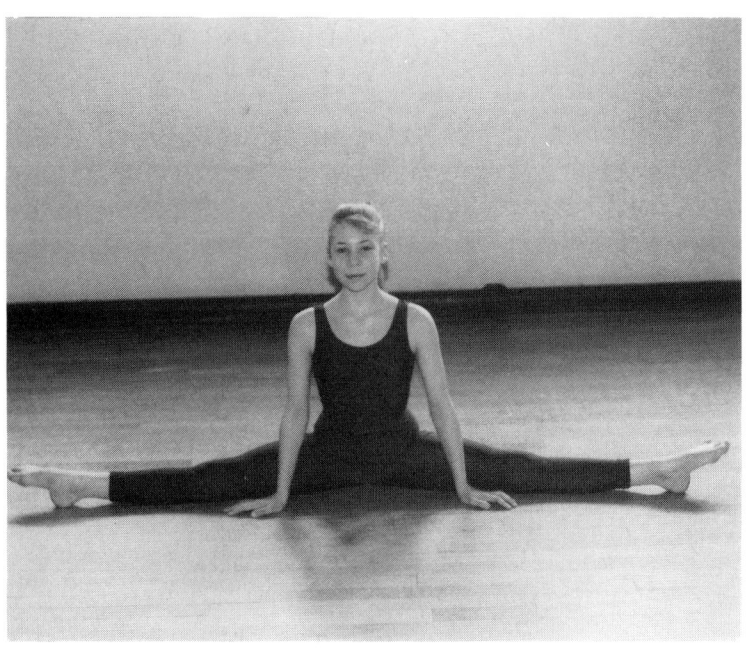

1 *Ease yourself down into the splits position.*

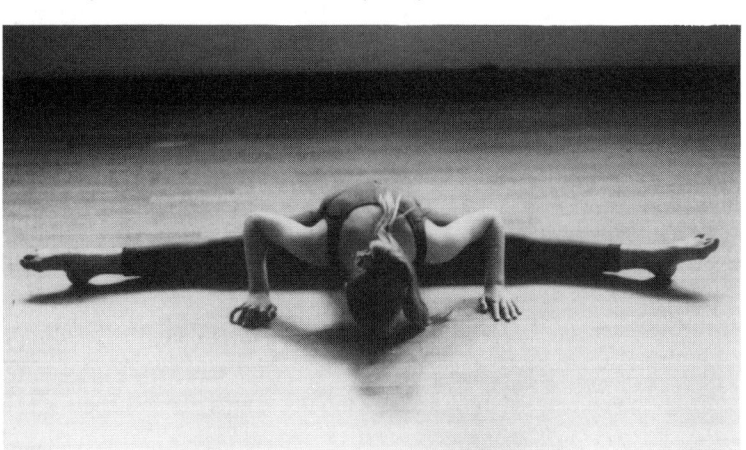

2 *Bend to the centre.*

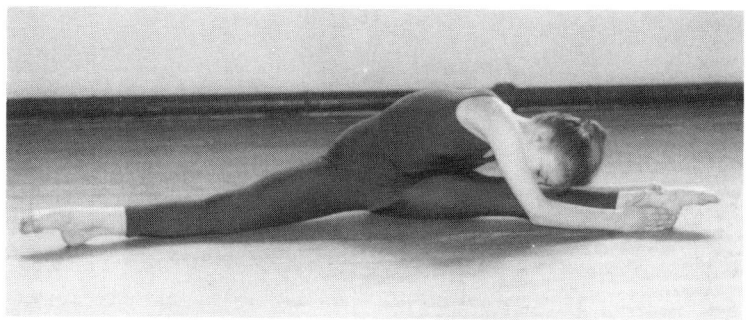

3 *Bend to the left.*

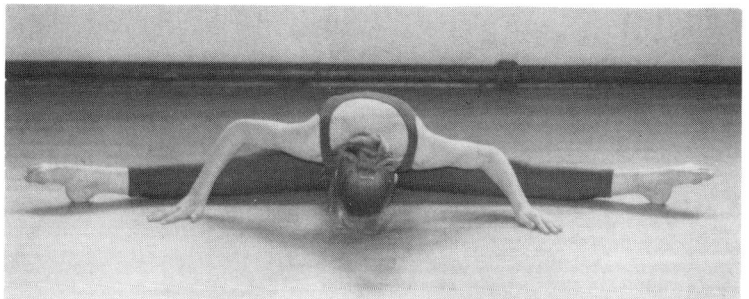

4 *Bend to the centre.*

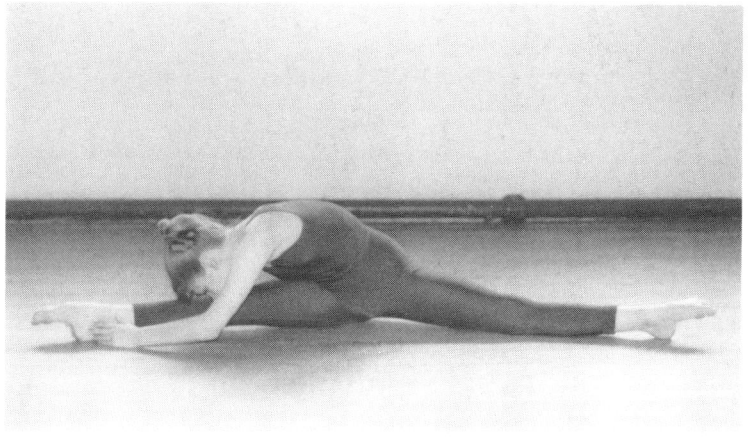

5 *Bend to the right.*

Splits II

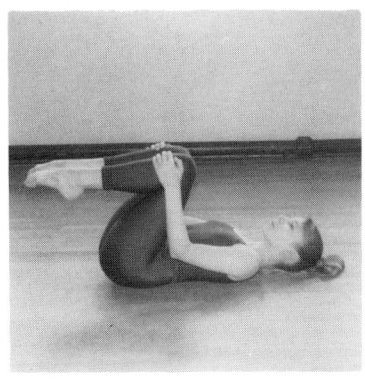 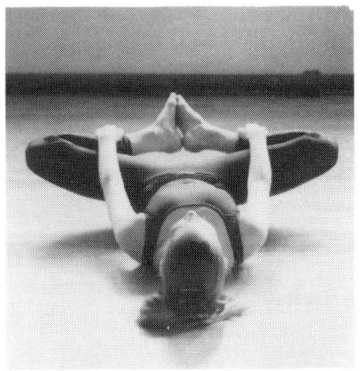

1 *Lie on your back and pull your knees up.*

2 *Let your knees drop and pull on your shins. Your feet should be pressed together.*

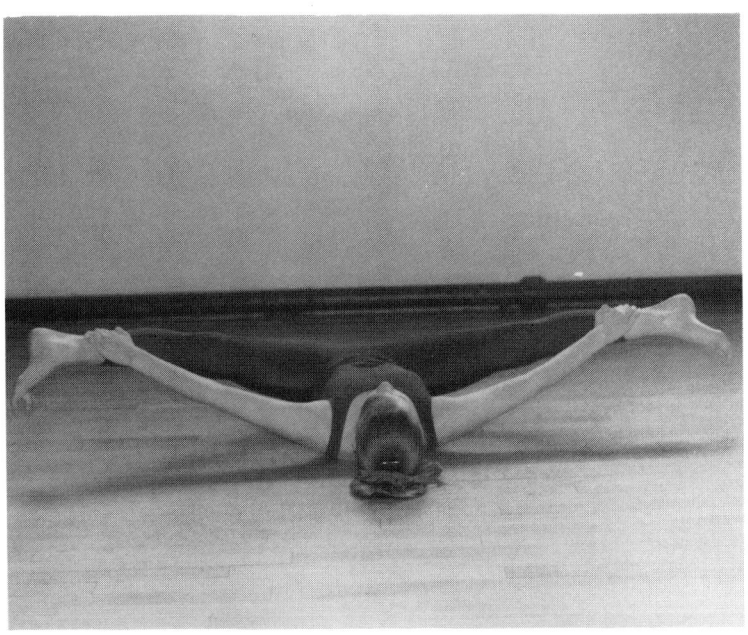

3 *Spread your legs and pull on your ankles. Return to starting position and repeat the exercise.*

Sit-Ups

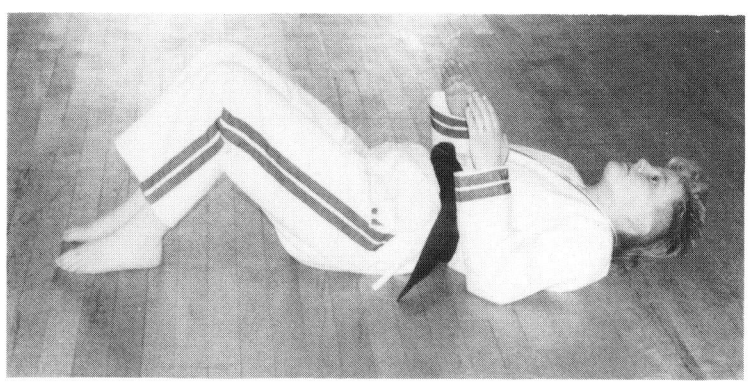

1 *Lie on your back with bent knees.*

2 *Sit a third of the way up and return to the starting position.*

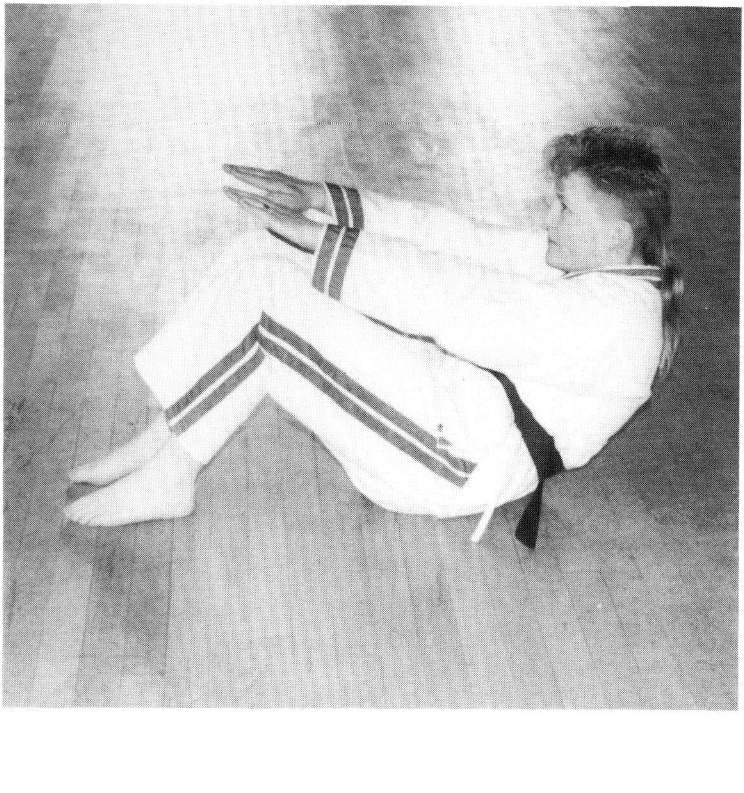

Press-Ups

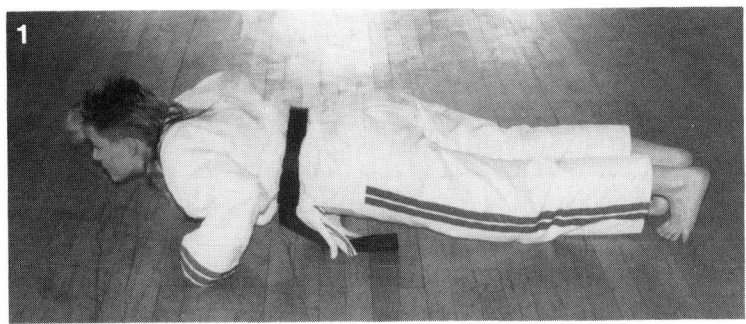

1 *Support yourself on your fists. Keep your body straight.*

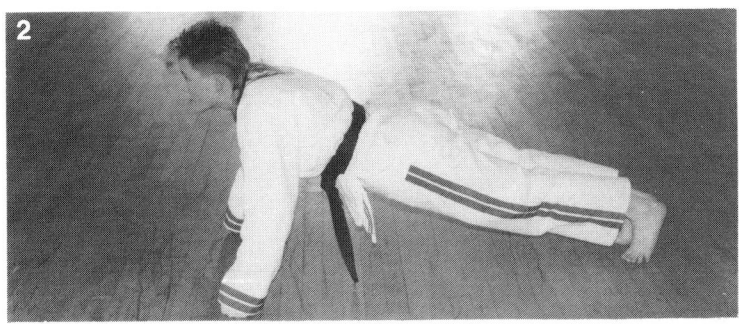

2 *Push yourself up without bending your body.*

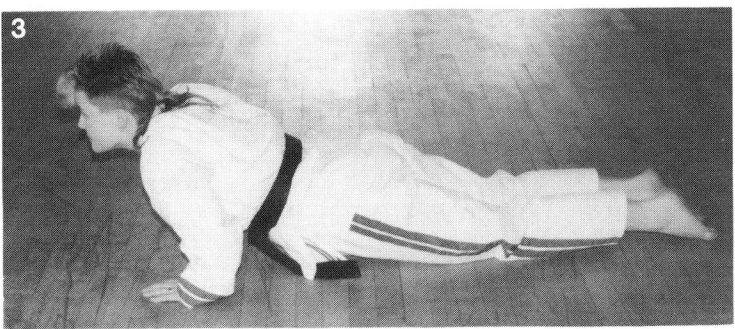

3 4 *If you find these press-ups too hard do them on your hands and knees.*

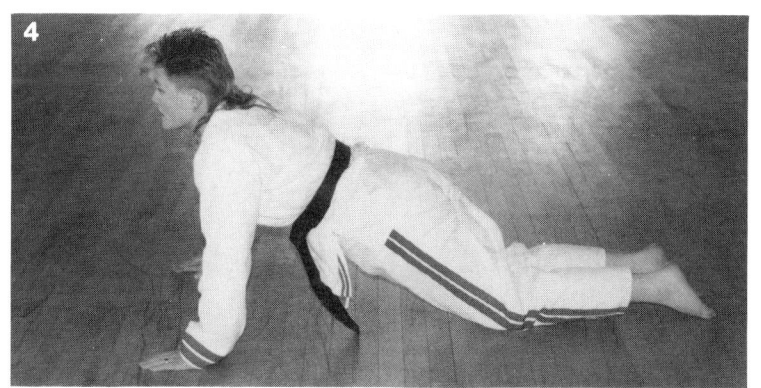

Back Stretch

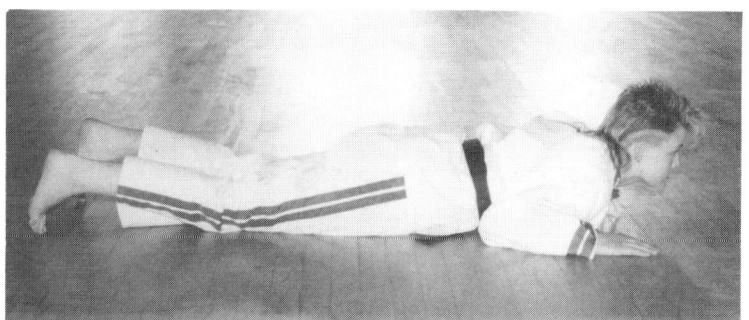

1 *Lie on your stomach*

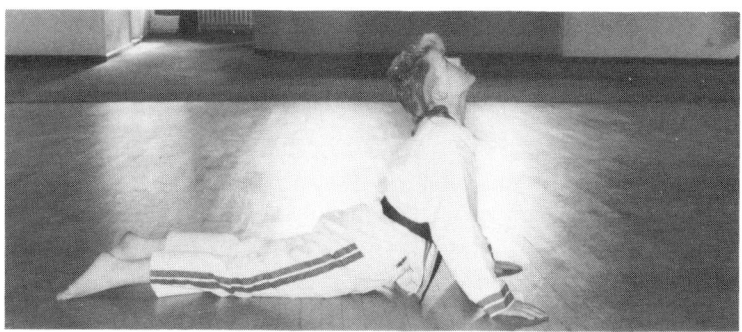

2 *Push yourself back keeping your hips pressed to the floor. Look up as you stretch.*

2

BASICS

It is essential to have a good foundation in basics and the essence of success is repetition. Human nature is in many respects fickle and most people show only bursts of enthusiasm for fads that come and go in their lives. Few experience the sense of achievement attainable after years of striving.

The sterling martial artist never neglects basics and he will perform them all his life, sometimes every day. The basic kicks, blocks, punches and strikes are the building blocks of any martial art. There is often controversy over minor points of technique among the different styles and unfortunately some instructors insist that their way is right to the exclusion of all others. Such an attitude is redolent of intolerance and even bigotry. Everybody has a unique bodytype and it is not a good thing to make all students conform to the same rigid, unbending discipline.

In martial dance, although integrity of martial arts technique is crucial, other factors come into play—high on the agenda are individualism and aesthetic self-expression. Hence there is more leeway for different ways of performing techniques. If a move 'feels' wrong to a dancer he is entitled to find his own way of performing it.

Practise at least some of these techniques every day. Many of them, especially the hand movements, can be performed in a confined area like the office or your front room. The techniques illustrated here have been selected because they have been utilized in the subsequent dance routines.

Hands

Left Jab

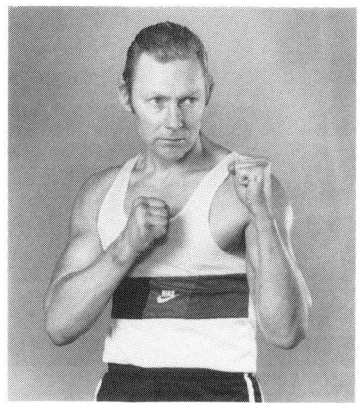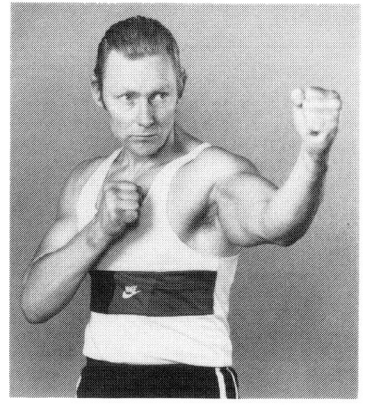

1 *Hold the left fist in the ready position.*

2 *Punch straight (and after full extension snap back the fist to starting position).*

Right Straight Punch

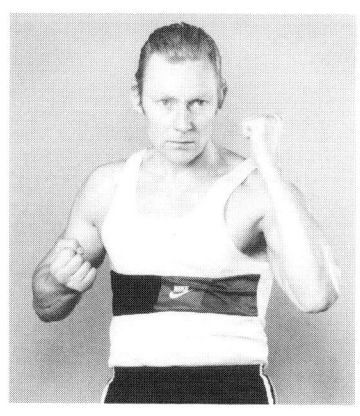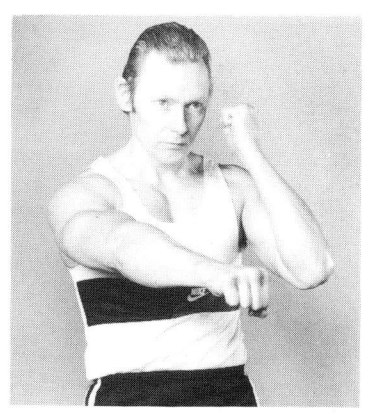

1 *Bring right fist back in ready position. The fist is turned upwards.*

2 *Drive the fist forward in a straight line turning it over at the point of full extension.*

Knifehand

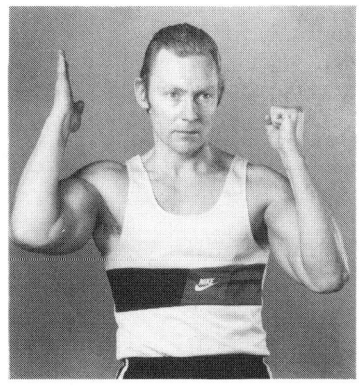 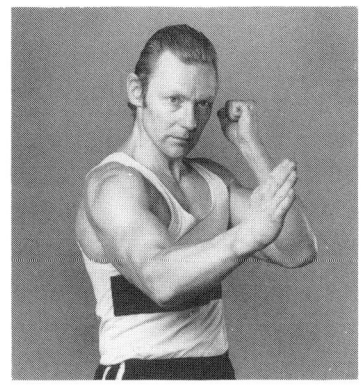

1 *With your right hand in a knifehand shape, raise it so that the palm faces your right ear.*

2 *Strike downwards keeping the fingers and thumb tightly closed.*

Ridgehand

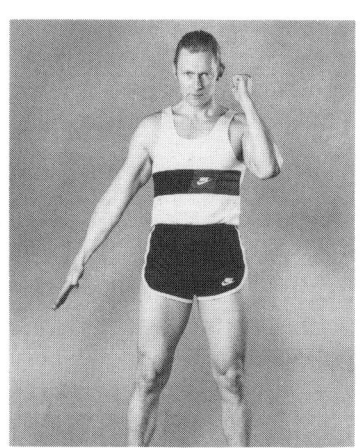 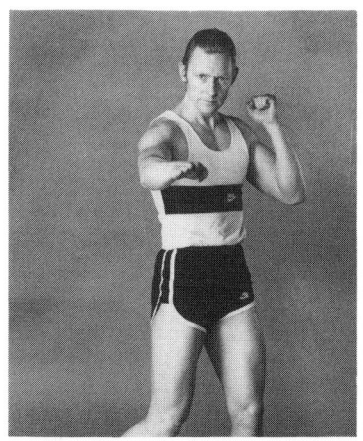

1 *Extend your right hand in a knifehand shape.*

2 *Strike up ridgehand — that is with the inside of the hand (knifehand uses the side of the hand opposite the thumb and ridgehand the thumb side).*

Hammerfist

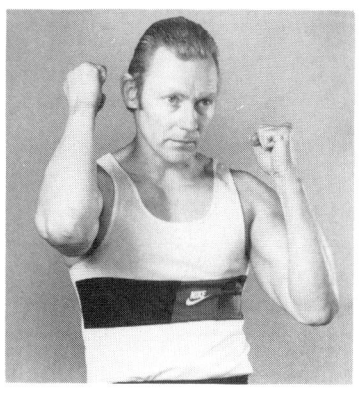 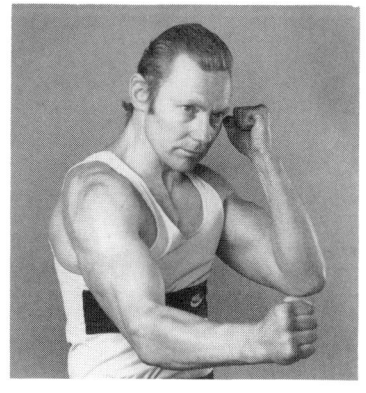

1 *Raise your right fist.*

2 *Strike down like a hammer with the bottom of the fist as the striking area.*

Elbow Strike — Inward

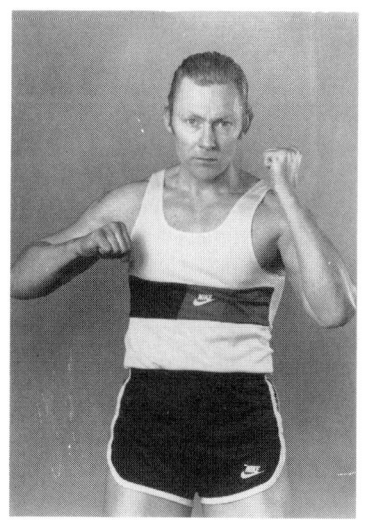 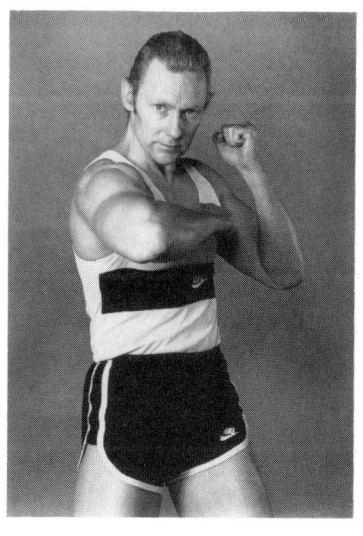

1 *Hold your right elbow up and out to your right.*

2 *Strike inwards to the centre.*

Elbow Strike — Outward

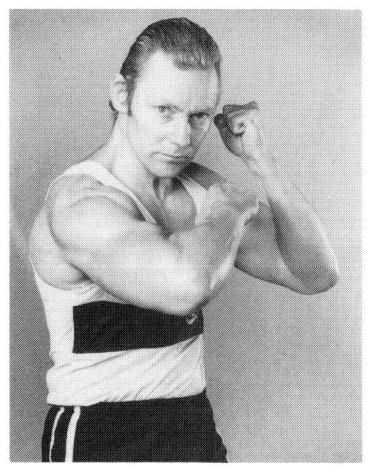 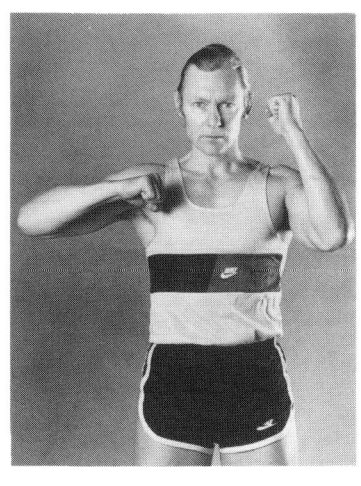

1 *Adopt the position of the last movement (2).*

2 *Strike outwards.*

Backfist

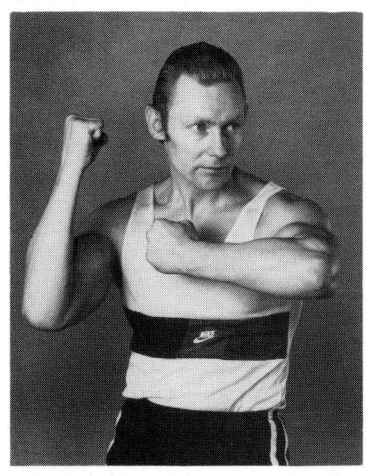 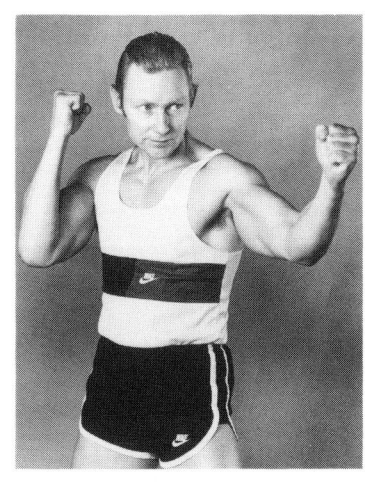

1 *Raise your left fist to your right shoulder.*

2 *Extend and strike with the back of the knuckles.*

Left Hook

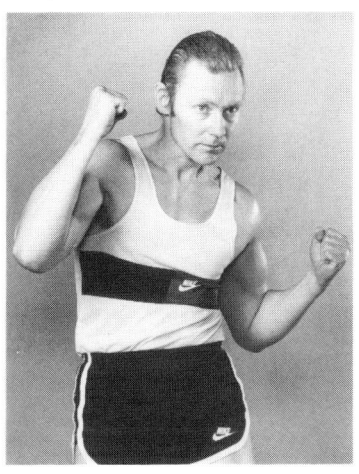 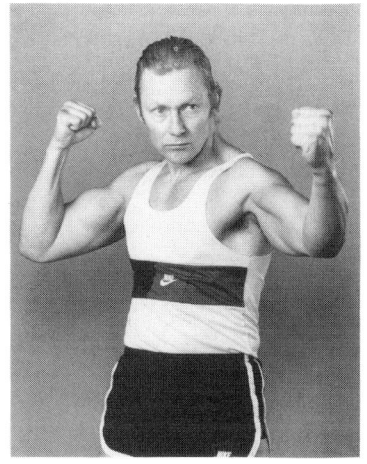

1 *Pull back your left shoulder.* **2** *Hook the punch round in a semicircle.*

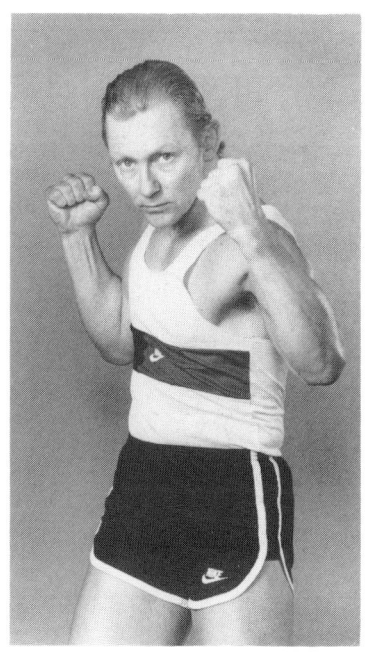

3 *Finishing point.*

Left Uppercut

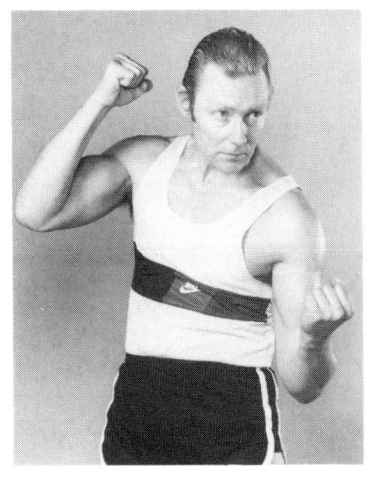
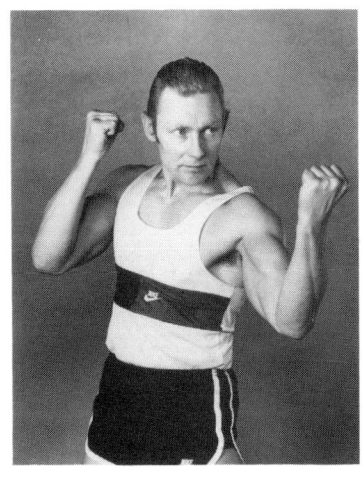

1 *Drop your left fist.*

2 *Drive it upwards.*

Rising Block

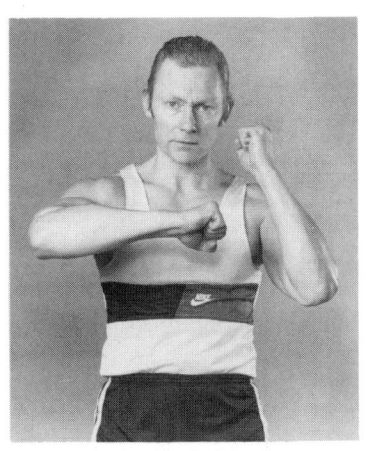
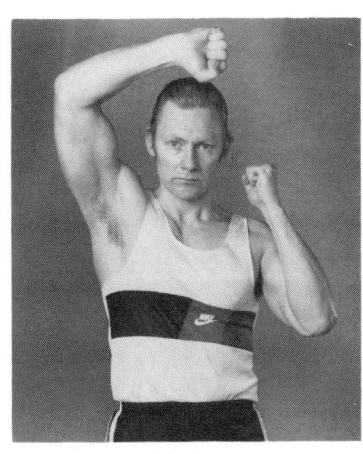

1 *Raise your right forearm into a horizontal position.*

2 *Thrust the forearm upwards, twisting the fist so that the palm faces out at the finishing point.*

Downward Block

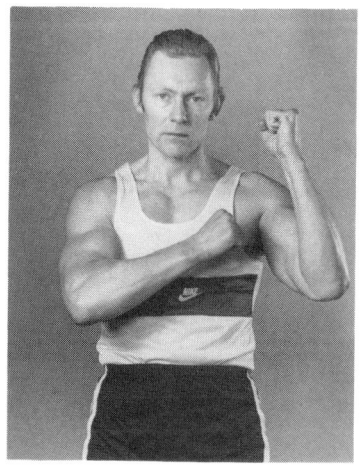 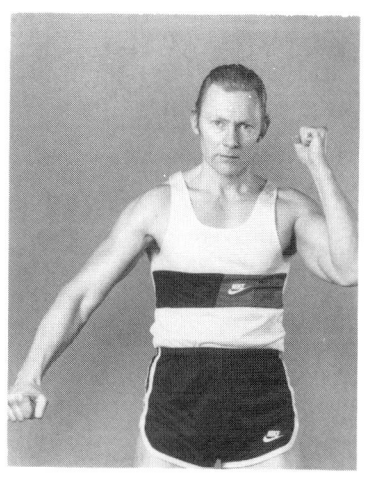

1 *Take your right arm across your body to your left shoulder.*

2 *Strike down and outwards.*

Inward Block

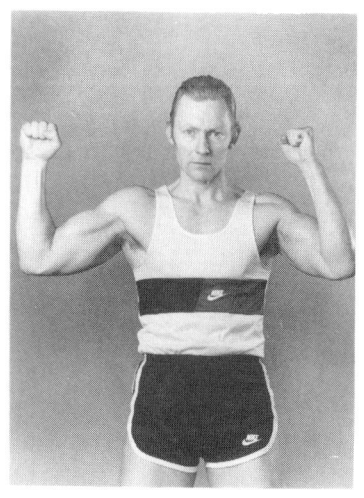 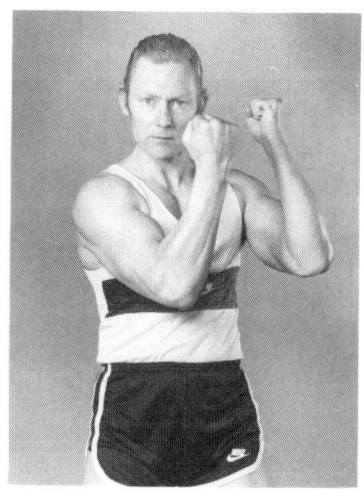

1 *Raise your right fist outwards.*

2 *Move the forearm across your body to its centre line.*

Outward Block

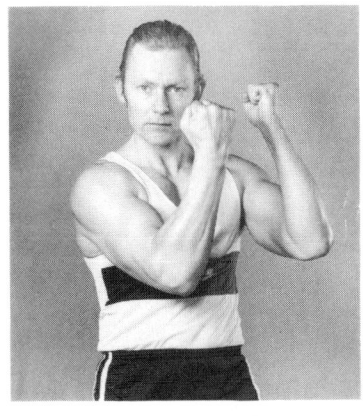 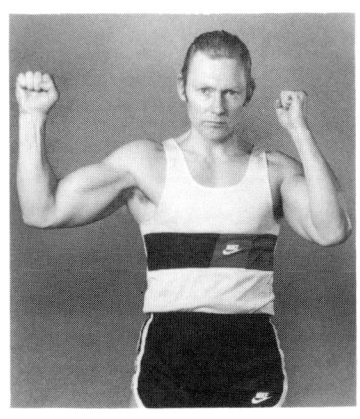

1 *Hold your fist up in front of you.*

2 *Strike outwards and turn the fist.*

Kicks

Frontkick

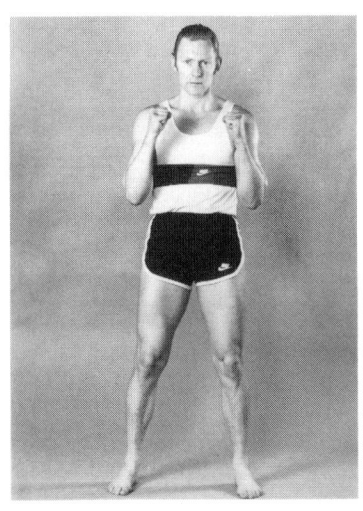 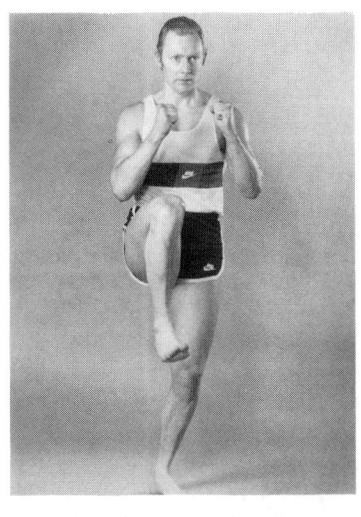

1 *Stand in ready position with guard*

2 *Raise your right knee straight in front of you.*

3 *Extend the lower leg.*

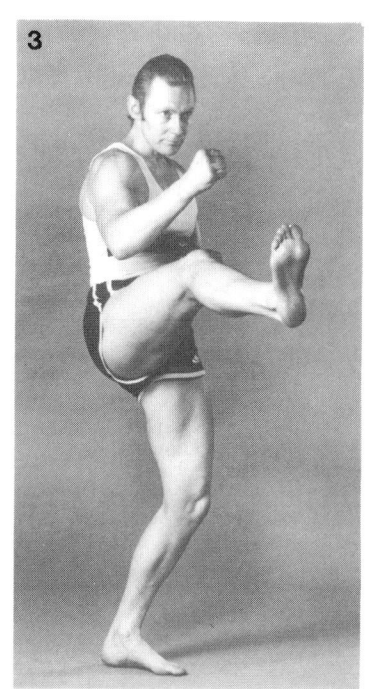

4 *Pull the kick back after full extension.*

5 *Return to ready position and repeat with the left leg.*

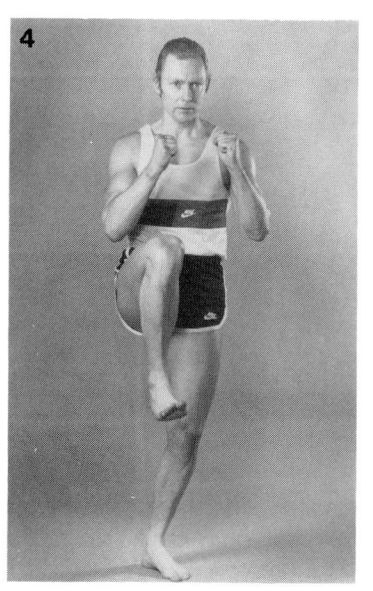

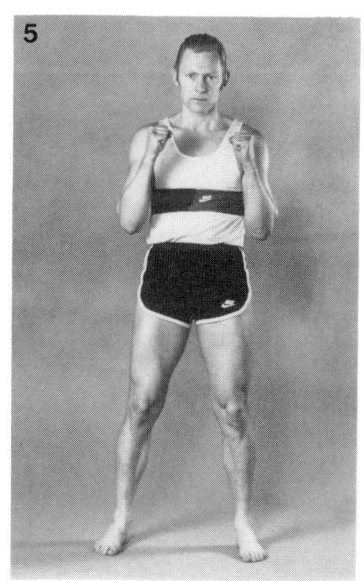

Roundhouse

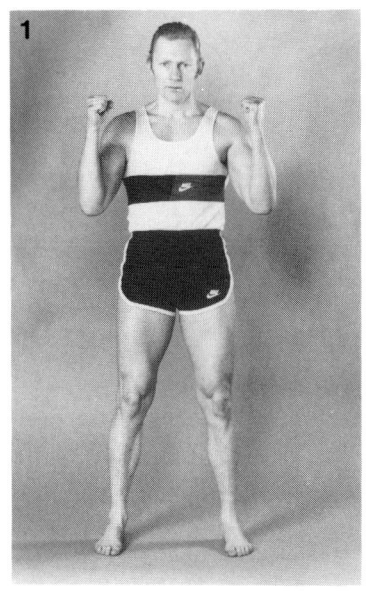

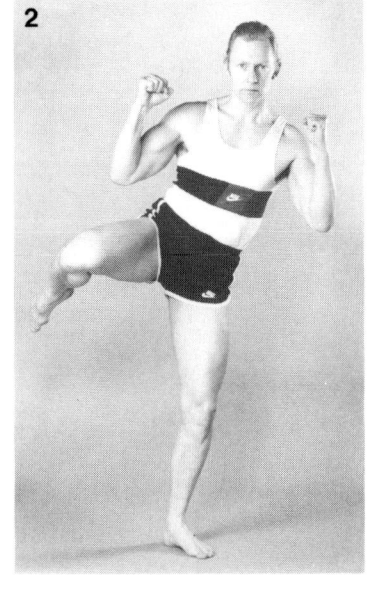

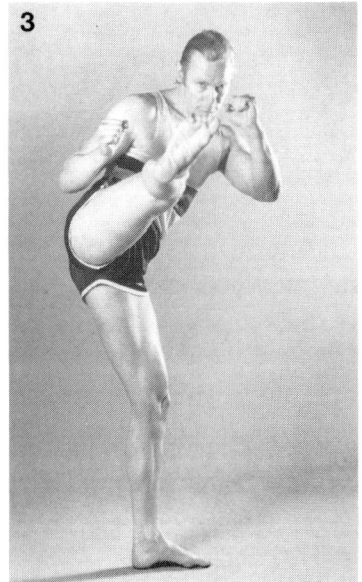

1 *Take up ready position.*

2 *Raise your knee outwards.*

3 *Extend the lower leg and turn the body so that the hip is thrust behind the kick.*

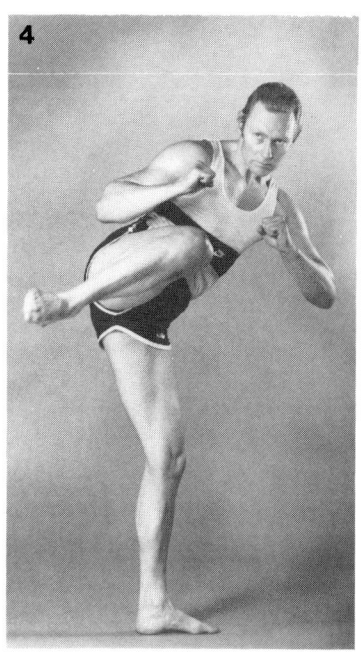

4 *Pull the kick back after full extension.*

5 *Return to starting position and repeat the kick with the left leg.*

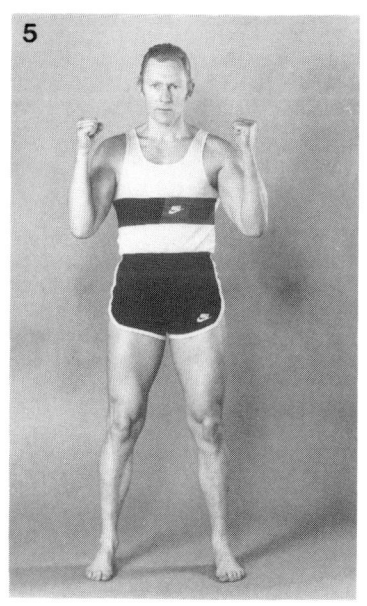

It is important to remember that if the body turns too much into the side-pn position while performing roundhouse it will be more difficult to keep to the beat of the music, so try to keep the body square-on or facing the target area you are kicking towards.

Crescent Kick

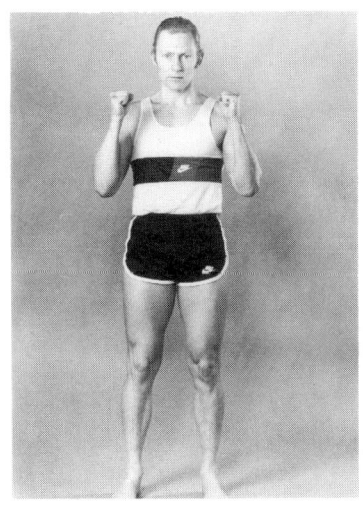

1 *Adopt the ready position.*

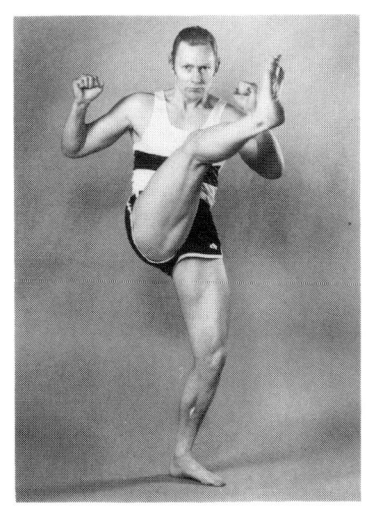

2 *Throw your right leg over to your left side.*

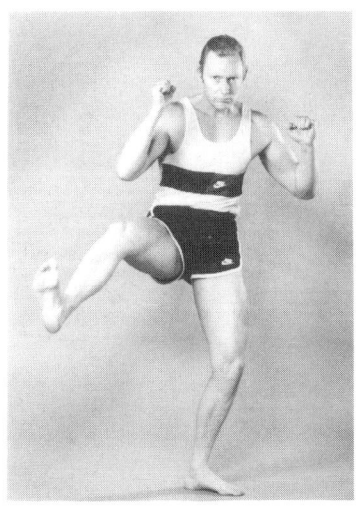

3 *Swing it round in a circular motion so that the foot passes in front of your face and down to your right.*

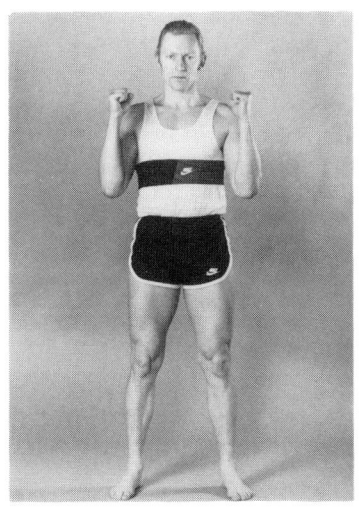

4 *Return to starting position and repeat the kick with the left leg.*

Knee Block

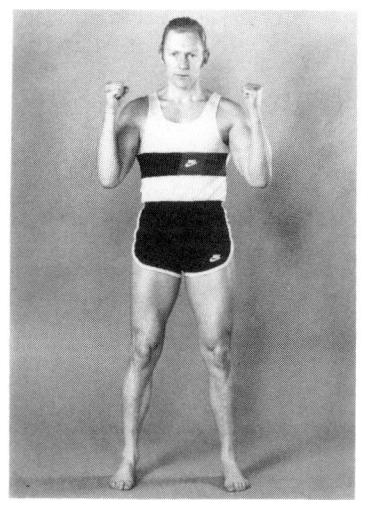

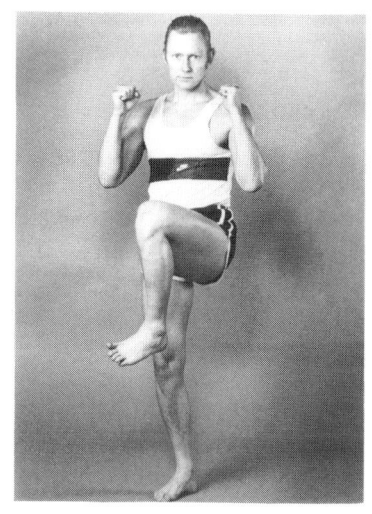

1 *Adopt the ready stance.*

2 *Raise the left knee across your body.*

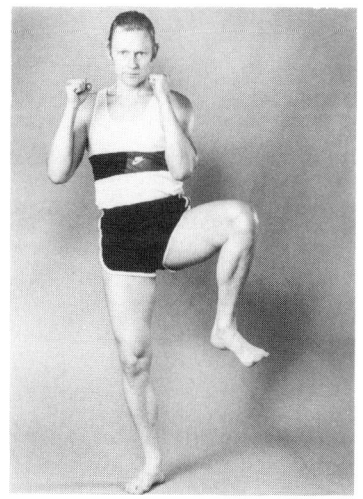

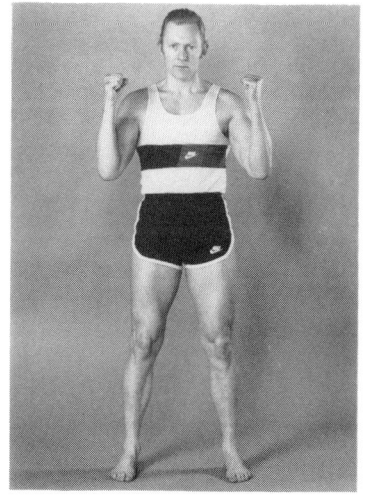

3 *Swing the knee to your outside left.*

4 *Return to the starting position and repeat with the right leg.*

Back-Kick

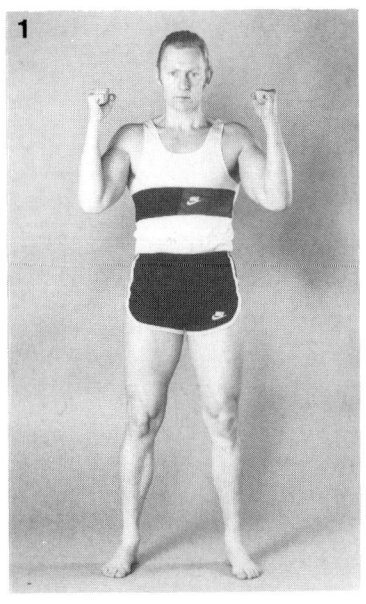

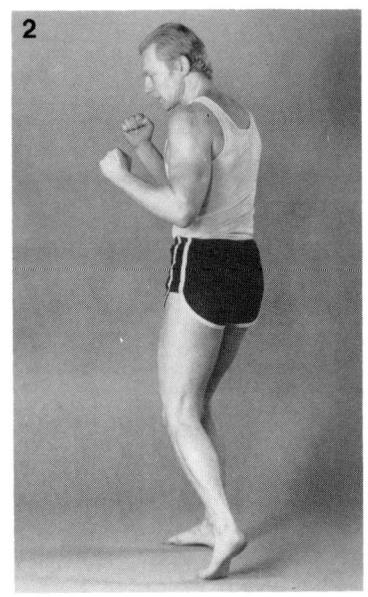

1 *Adopt the ready position.*

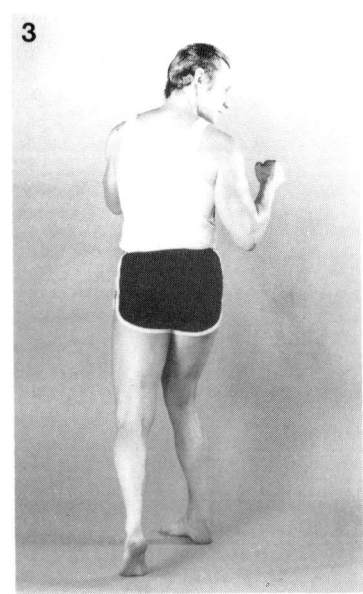

2 3 *Turn round towards your right, moving your right foot across so that it ends up in front of the left.*

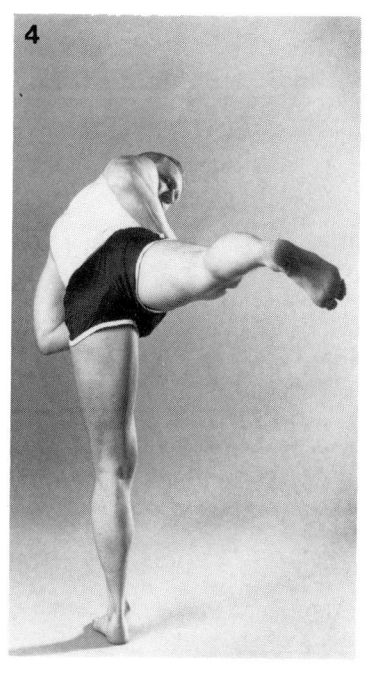

4 *Kick straight back with the heel.*

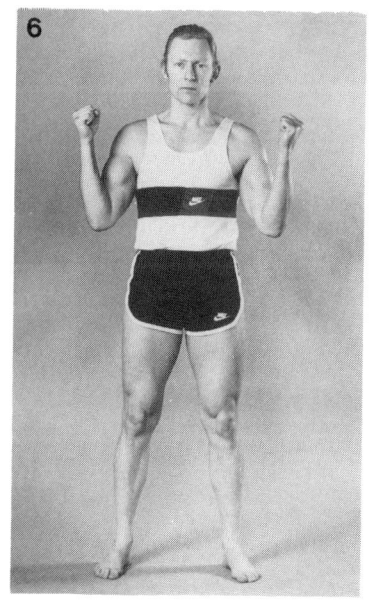

5 *Bring back the kick.*

6 *Return to starting position and repeat with the left leg.*

Hook-Kick

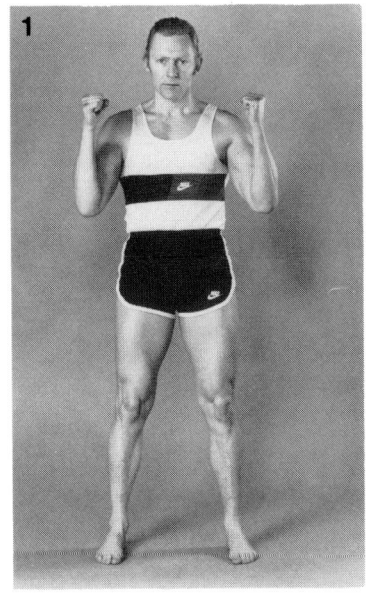

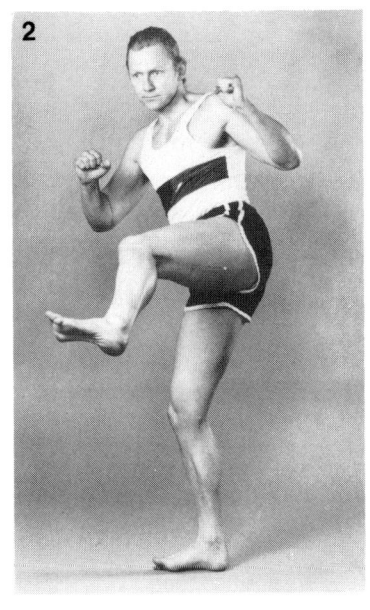

1 *Adopt a ready position.*

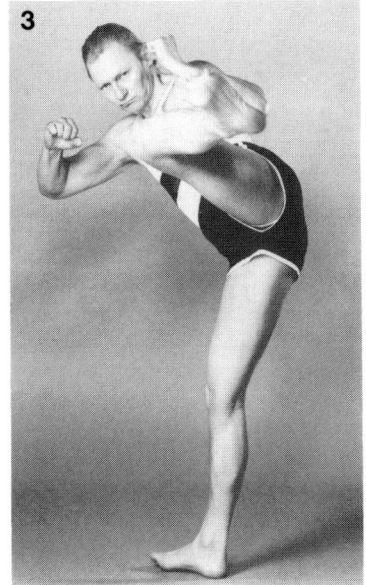

2 *Throw the left leg over to your right.*

3 *Hook it back in a circular motion striking with the heel.*

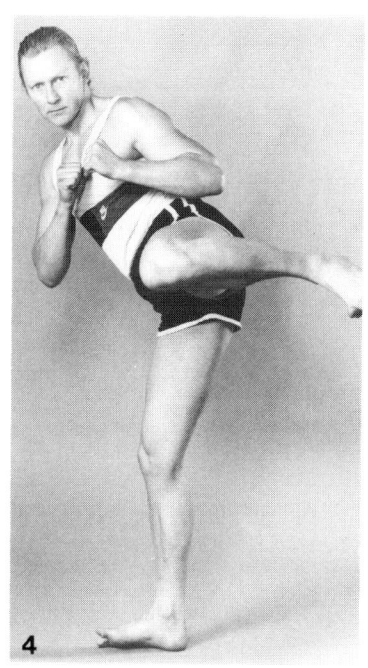

4 *Pull the kick back.*

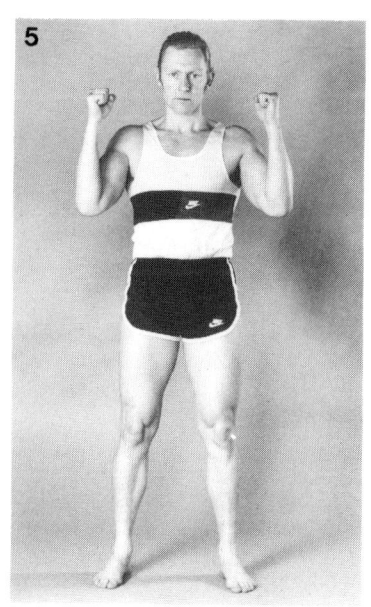

5 *Return to starting position and repeat with the right leg.*

3

AEROBICS

Training to music is fun and inspiring. Music gives you energy. Martial aerobics are for stamina and fitness and you will find that performing these kicking combinations continuously for the duration of a record or two can be very tiring but will improve your kicking ability. The emphasis in this selection of martial aerobic exercises is on the kicks because using your feet in martial dance is so important and one can never get enough practice.

Squat Kicks

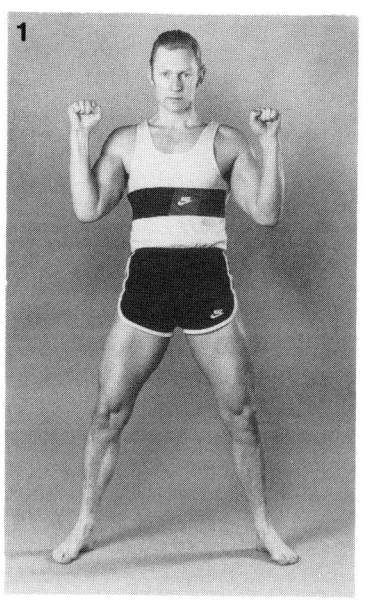

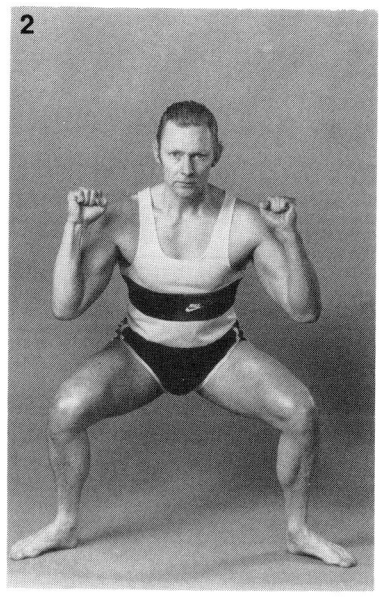

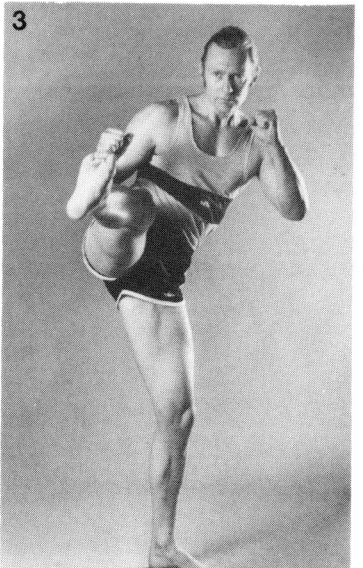

1 *Stand in a ready position.*

2 *Squat with hands in a guard position.*

3 *Stand and perform right roundhouse.*

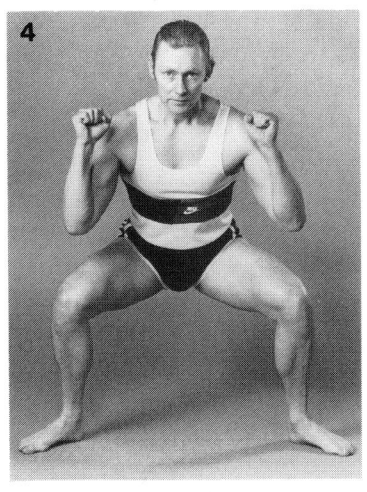

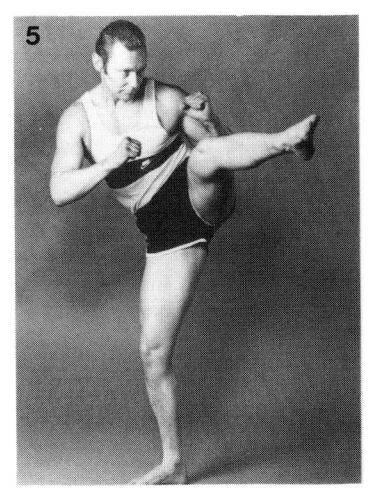

4 *Squat with hands in guard position.*

5 *Stand and perform left roundhouse.*

Sway kicks

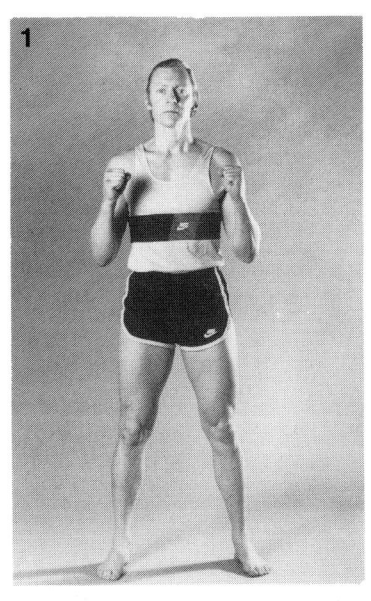

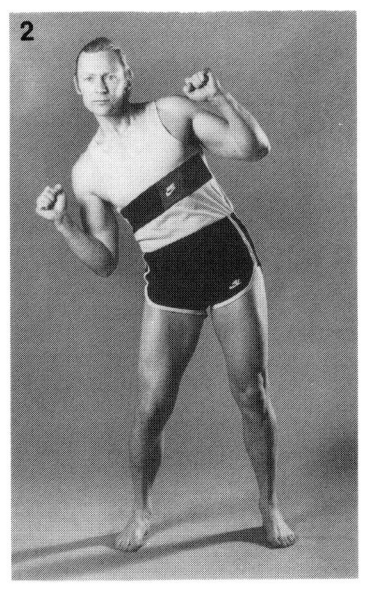

1 *Adopt a ready position.*

2 *Sway to the right.*

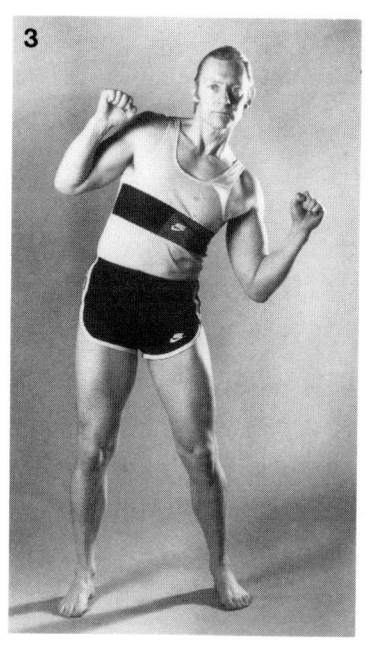 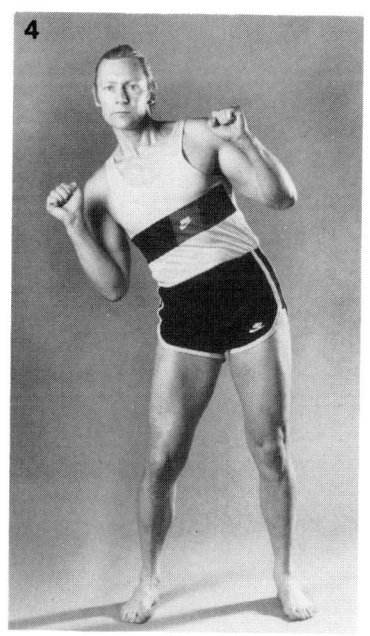

3 *Sway to the left.*

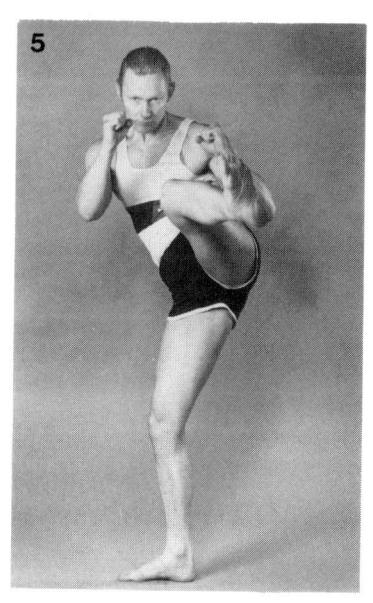

4 *Sway to the right.*

5 *Kick left roundhouse.*

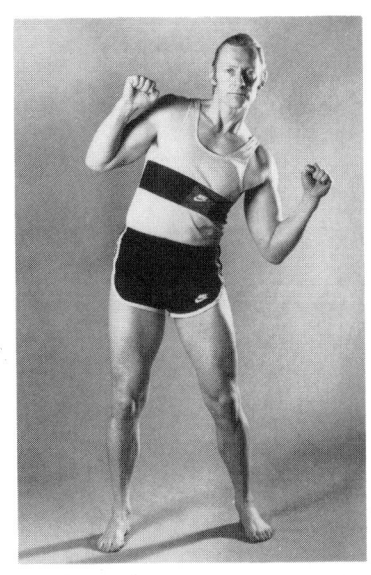

6 *Sway to the left.*

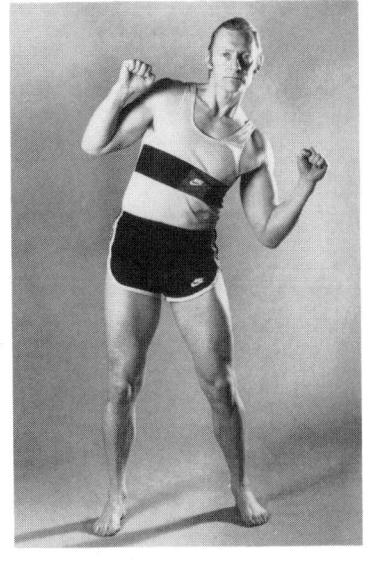

7 *Sway to the right.*

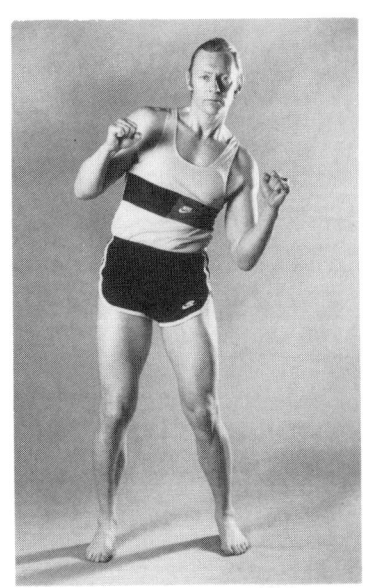

8 *Sway to the left.*

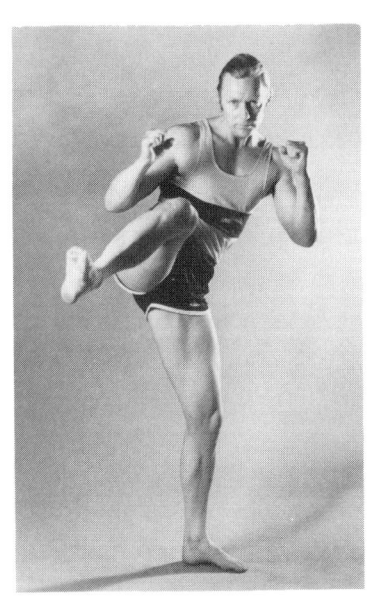

9 *Kick right roundhouse.*

Skip-Punching
An exercise in hand/foot co-ordination

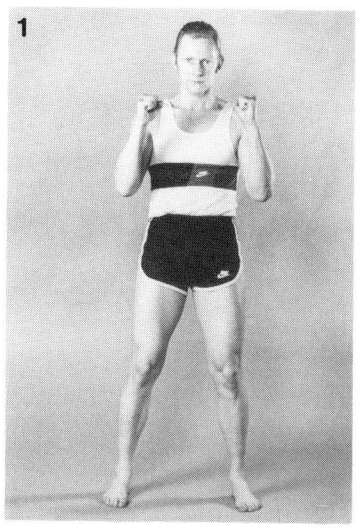

1 *Assume a ready position.*

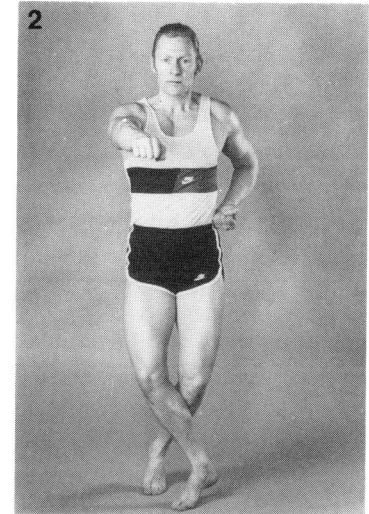

2 *Skip right leg over left and punch simultaneously with a right straight punch.*

3 *Skip out still holding the punch extended.*

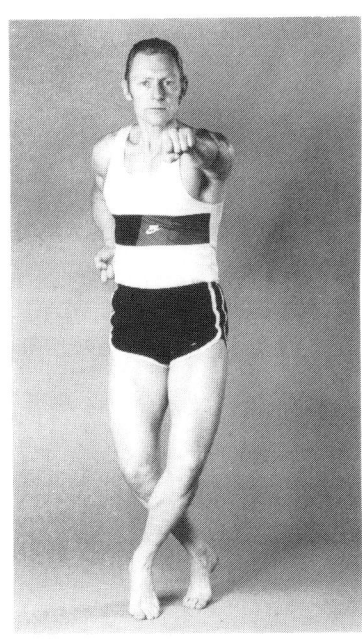

4 *Skip left leg over right while punching with the left.*

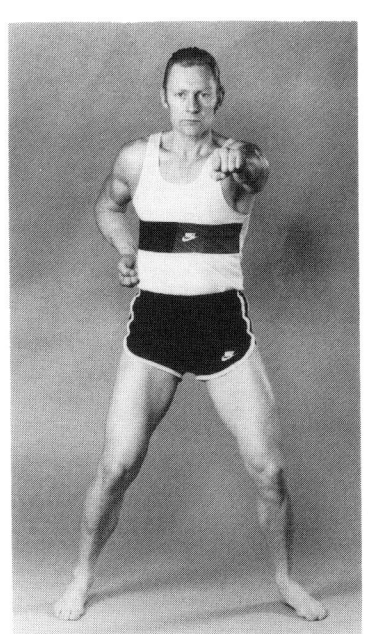

5 *Skip out holding the punch extended.*

Double Kicks
To be performed alternately with BOTH legs

Roundhouse/Back-Kick

1 *Stand with guard. (All double kicks performed from this stance).*

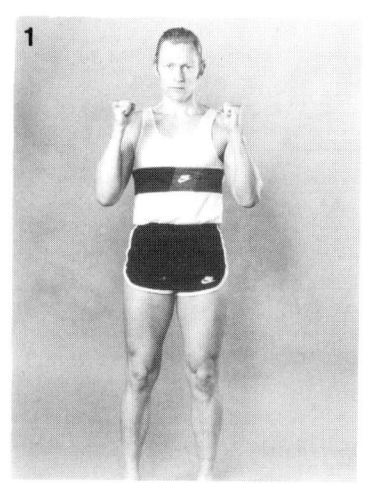

2 *Kick roundhouse with your right leg.*

3 *Put your foot down and immediately kick back-kick with the same leg. Repeat both kicks with the left leg.*

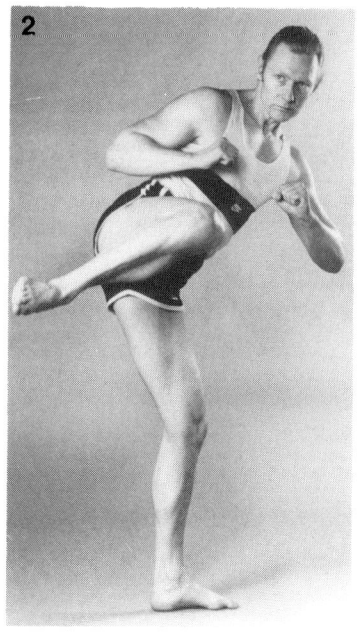

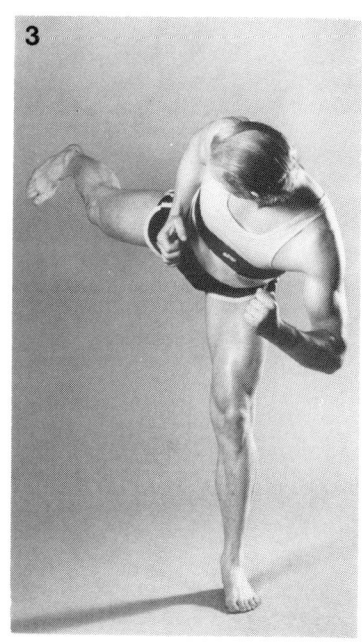

Double Roundhouse

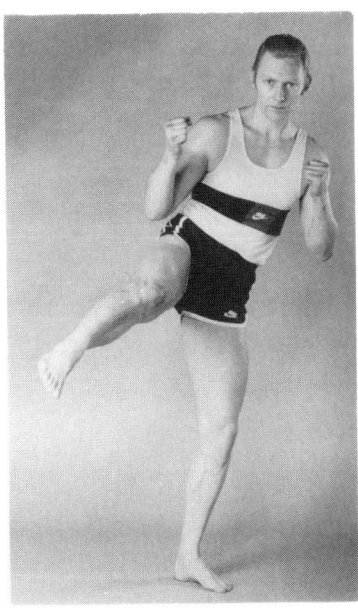

1 *Kick a low roundhouse with the right leg.*

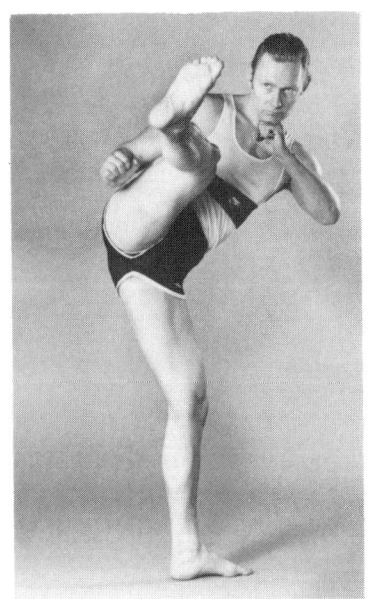

2 *Put your foot down and immediately perform another roundhouse kick but make it higher. Repeat both kicks with the left leg.*

Roundhouse/Knee Block

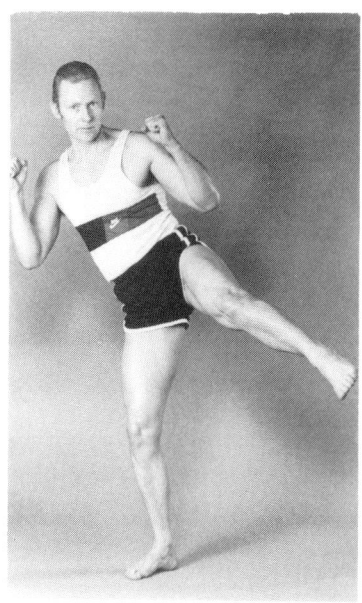

1 *Perform a low roundhouse kick with the left leg.*

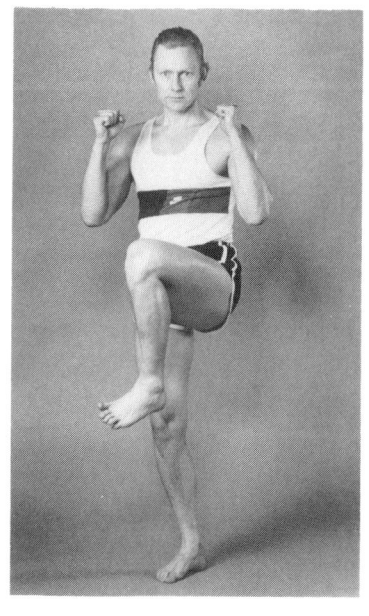

2 *Put your foot down and immediately perform a knee block with the same leg. Repeat both techniques with the right leg.*

Front-Kick/Roundhouse

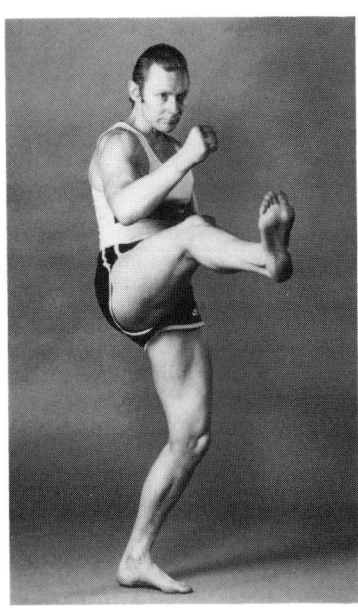

1 *Kick front-kick with the right leg.*

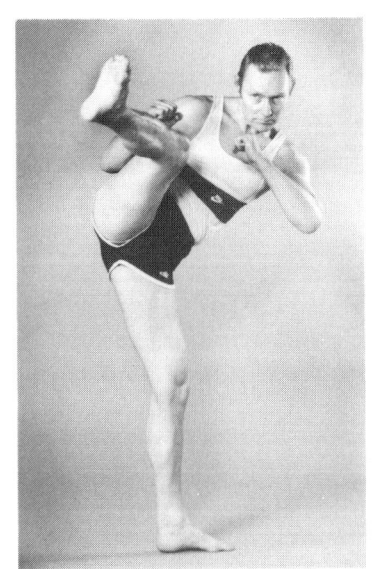

2 *Put your foot down and immediately kick roundhouse. Repeat kicks with the left leg.*

Roundhouse/Crescent Kick

1 *Kick roundhouse with the right leg.*

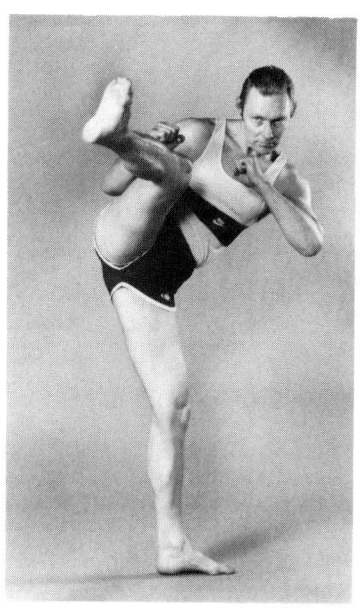

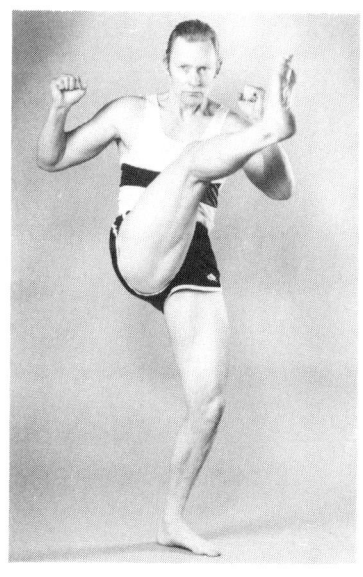

2 *Touch the foot down and immediately kick crescent kick. Repeat kicks with the left leg.*

4

ON-THE-SPOT ROUTINES

These routines are a test of hand and foot co-ordination. Try them to different records and different types of music with varied tempos. They probably work best with pop. After they become automatic you should progress to the stage where you can 'dance' them instead of going through the motions. Perform them in different directions, turning on the spot.

Routine One
Incorporating knifehand, knee block, and crescent kick.

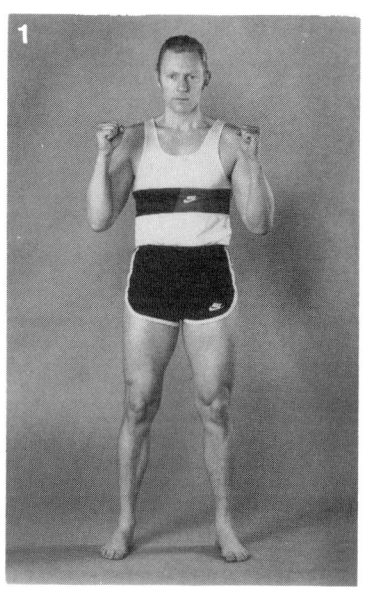

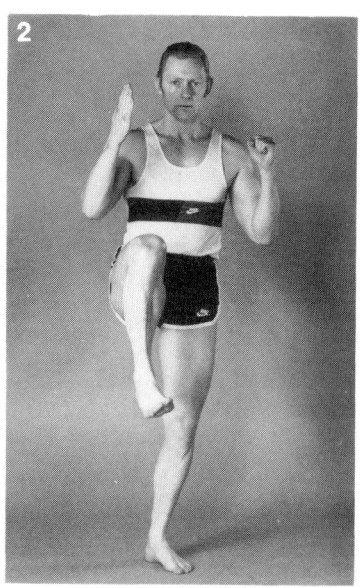

1 *Ready position.*

2 *Raise your right knee and lightly skim it with a ridgehand uppercut.*

3 *As the foot touches the ground perform an outward elbow strike.*

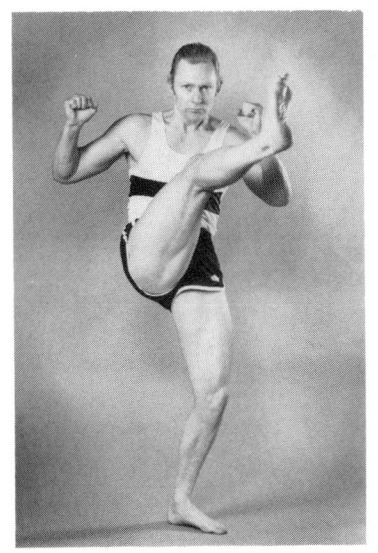 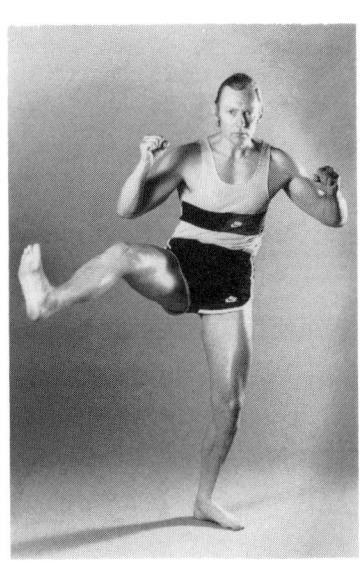

4 5 *Perform a crescent kick.*

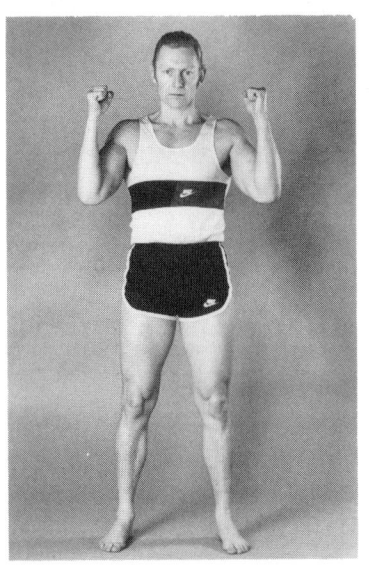

6 *Return briefly to ready position.*

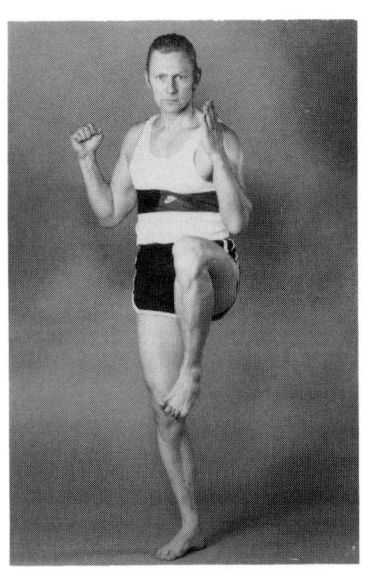

7 *Commence identical routine with the left side of your body.*

Routine Two
Incorporating knifehand, ridgehand, and front-kick

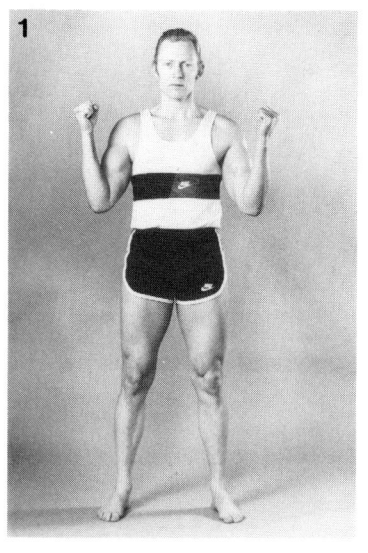

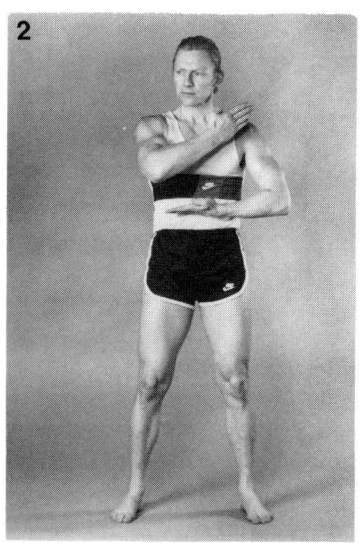

1 *Ready position*

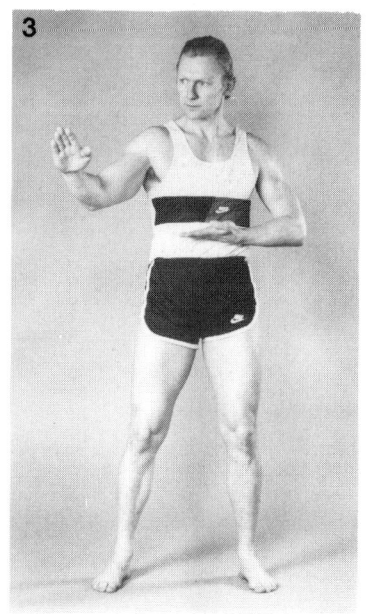

2 *Make a knifehand shape with both hands — the right with your palm facing your left shoulder, the left hand over your stomach.*

3 *Strike knifehand with the right hand at 45°.*

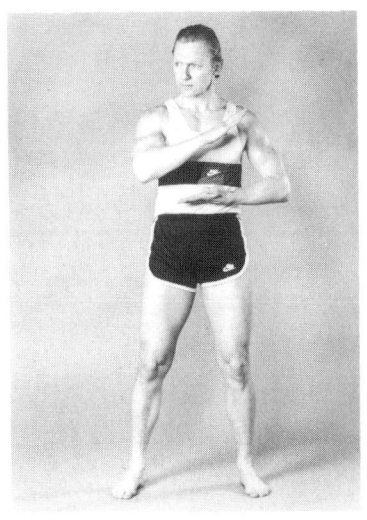

4 *Bring it back.*

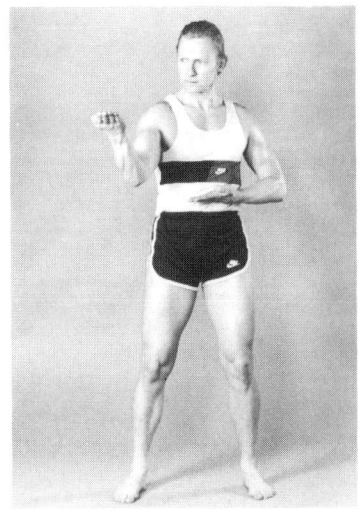

5 *Flip the hand over so the palm is facing upwards and strike ridgehand at 45°.*

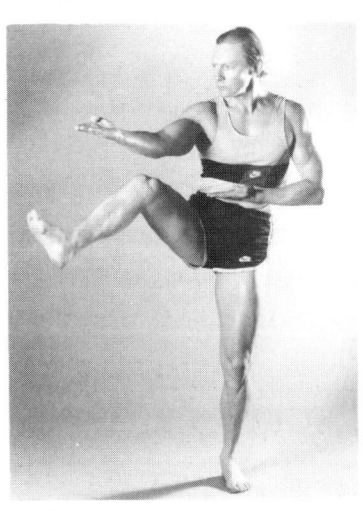

6 *Maintaining your hand positions, kick front-kick* **twice**. *Do not put your foot down between the kicks.*

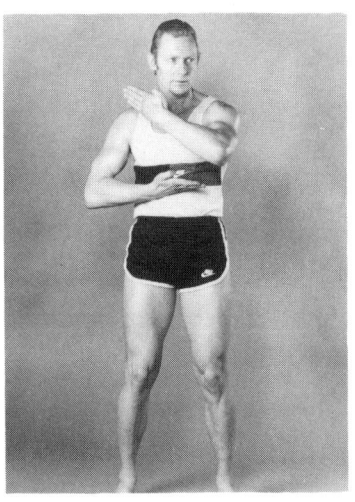

7 *Repeat the routine on the other side.*

Routine Three
Incorporating knifehand, ridgehand, and roundhouse.

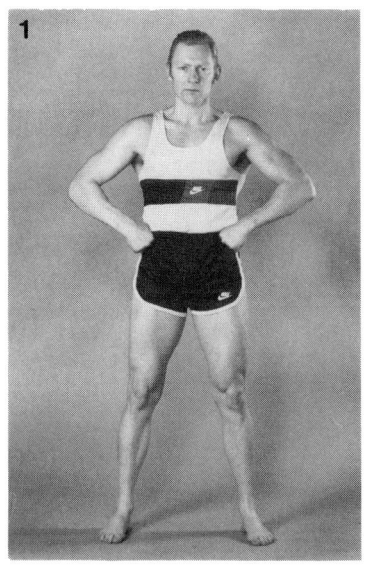

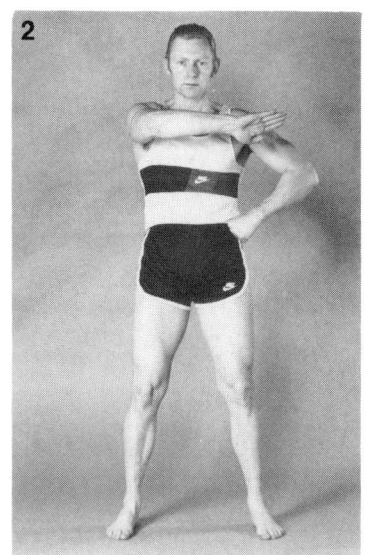

1 *Ready position with fists on hips.*

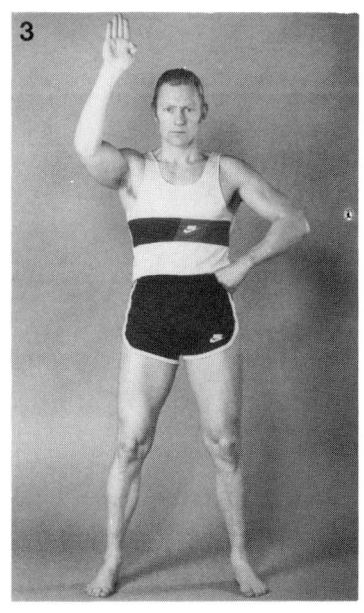

2 *Make a knifehand, shape with your right hand and take it to your left shoulder, turning it so you can see the back of the hand.*

3 *Take it over your head.*

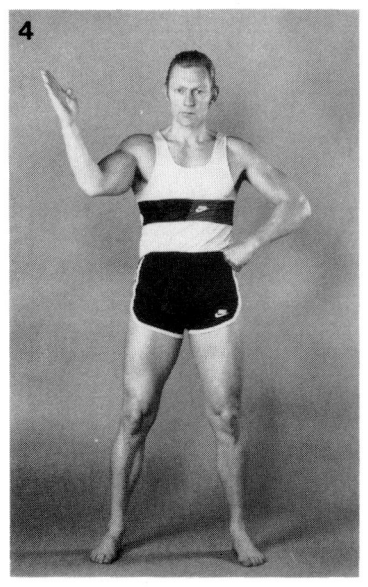

4 *Strike knifehand.*

5 6 7 *Repeat with your left hand.*

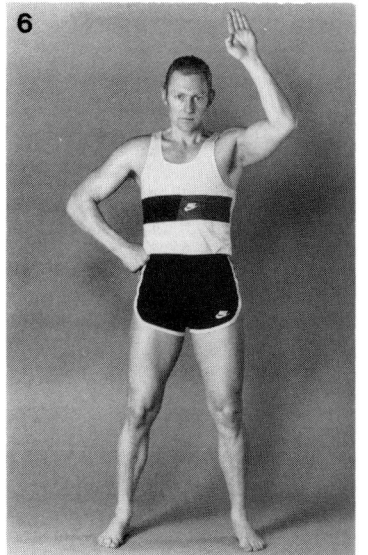

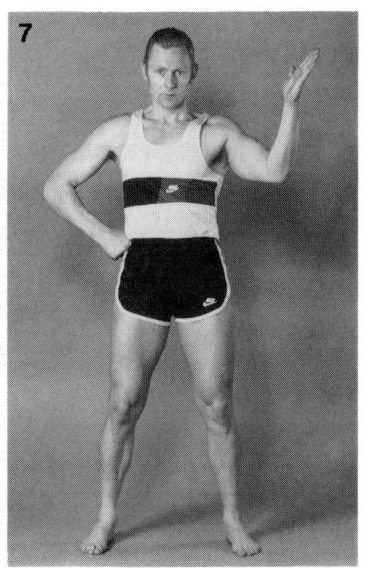

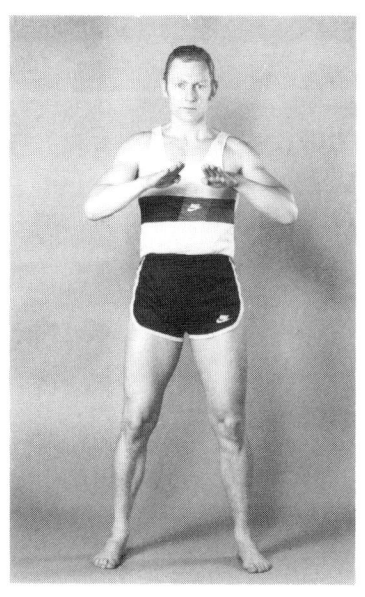

8 *Bring your hands in front of your chest with the palms facing down.*

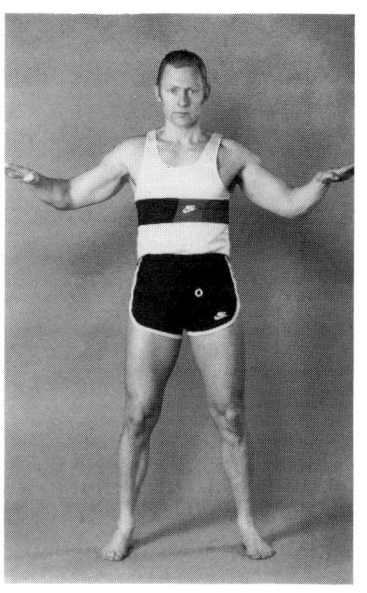

9 *Perform double knifehand strike.*

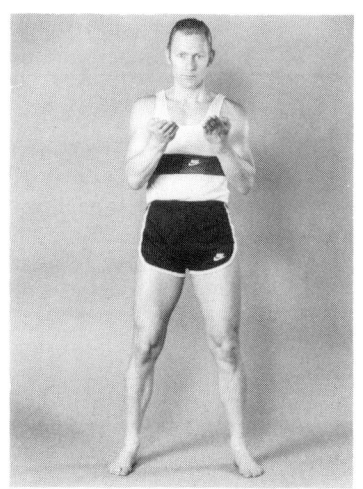

10 *Bring your hands back and turn your palms up.*

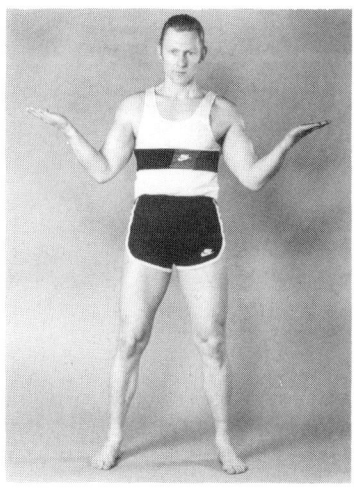

11 *Perform double strike ridgehand.*

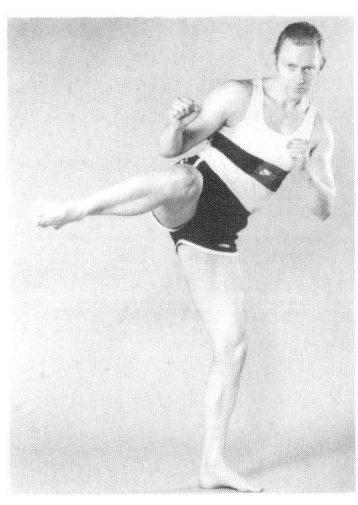 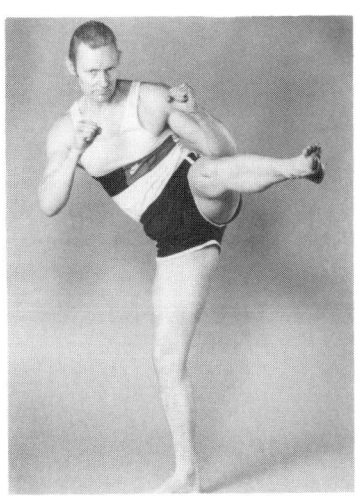

12 *Perform two roundhouse kicks with the right leg without putting your foot down in between kicks.*

13 *Perform two roundhouse kicks with the left leg. These roundhouse kicks can be on the same level or at different levels for the more advanced student (i.e. the first one low and the second one as high as you can get it).*

Routine Four
Incorporating elbow strike, four blocks, and hook kick.

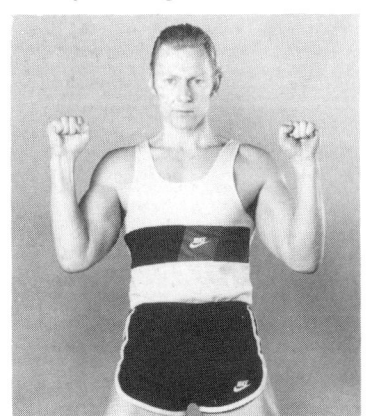

1 *Take up the ready position. (All the following hand techniques are performed with the same hand and without a pause).*

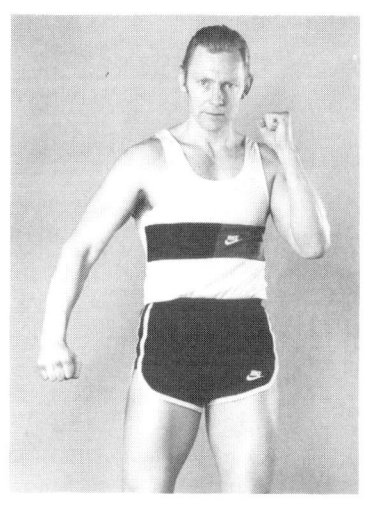

2 *Perform a downward block with your right hand.*

3 *Perform an outward block.*

4 *Perform an inward block.*

5 *Perform a rising block.*

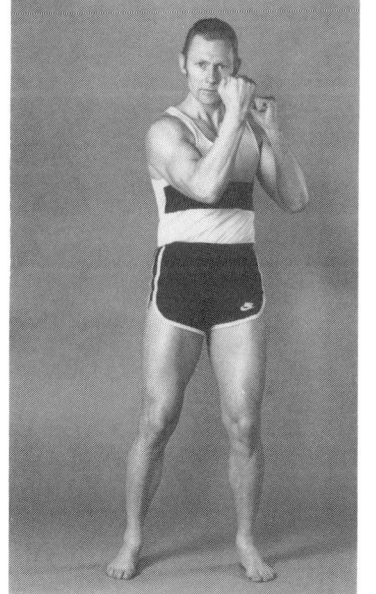

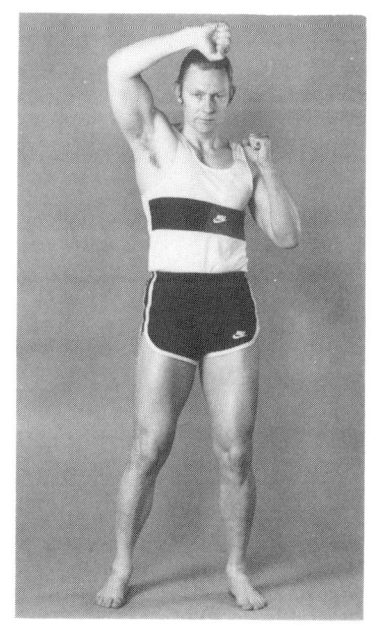

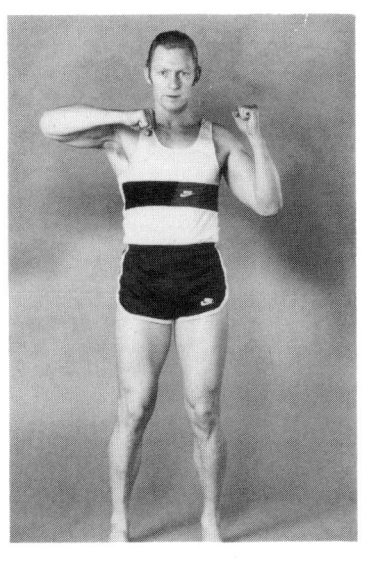

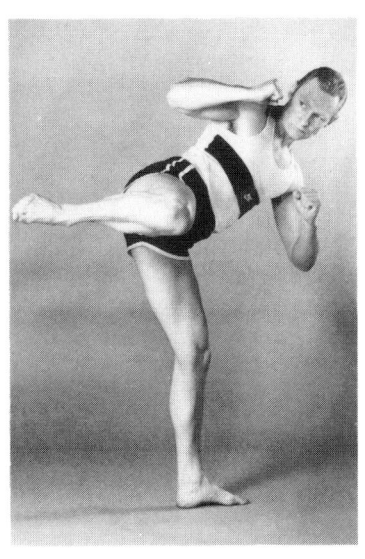

6 *Perform outward elbow strike.*

7 *Perform hook kick with the right leg. Repeat all the techniques on the left side, beginning with left downward block.*

Routine Five

Incorporating roundhouse, hook punch, uppercut, front-kick, and back-kick.

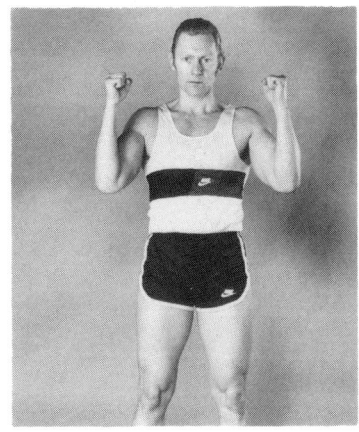

1 *Adopt ready position.*

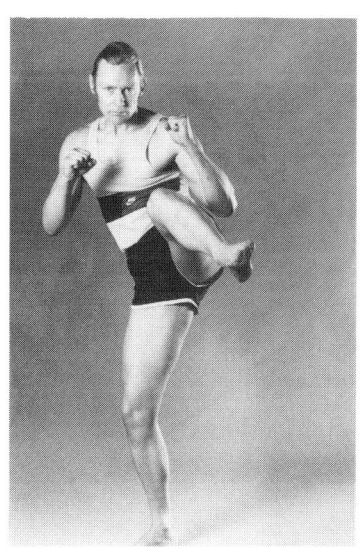 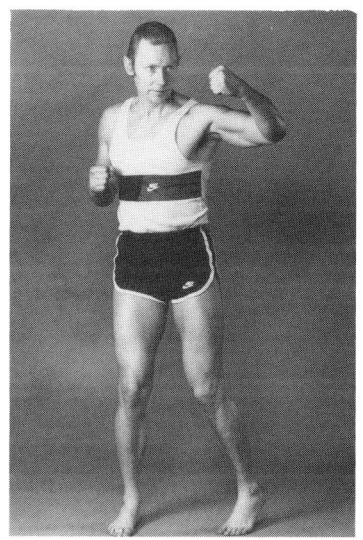

2 *Perform a left roundhouse.*

3 *As your foot touches the floor punch with a left hook.*

4 *Punch uppercut with the right hand.*

5 *Perform a right front-kick.*

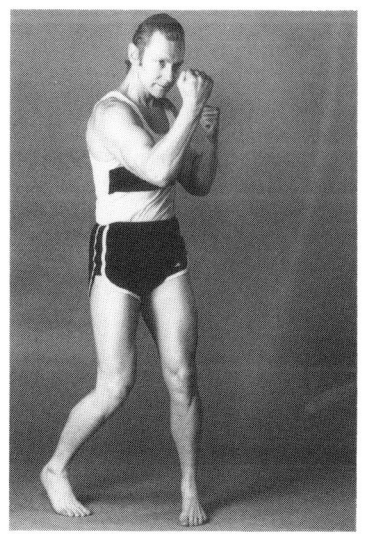 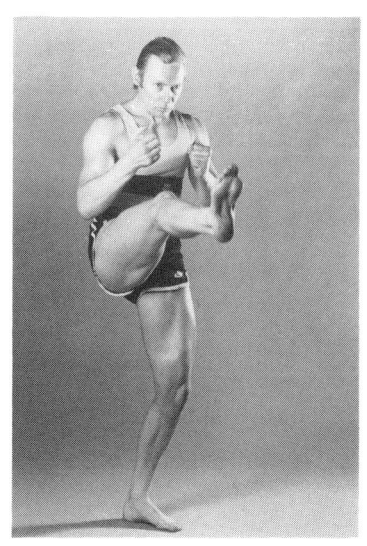

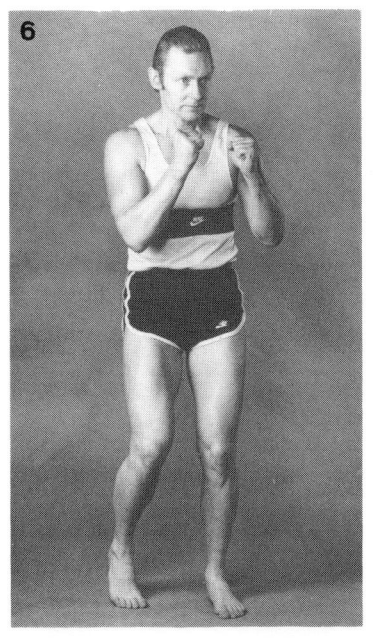

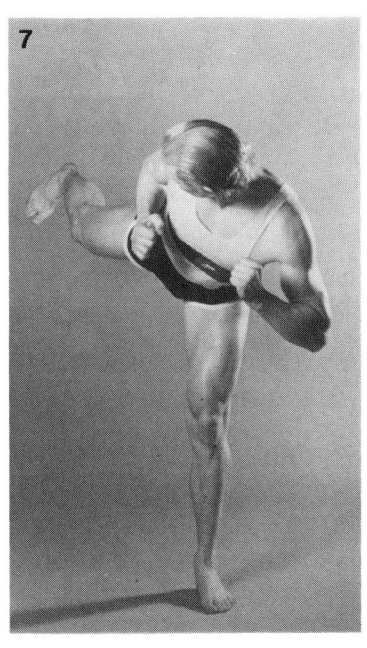

6 *Touch down with the kicking foot.*

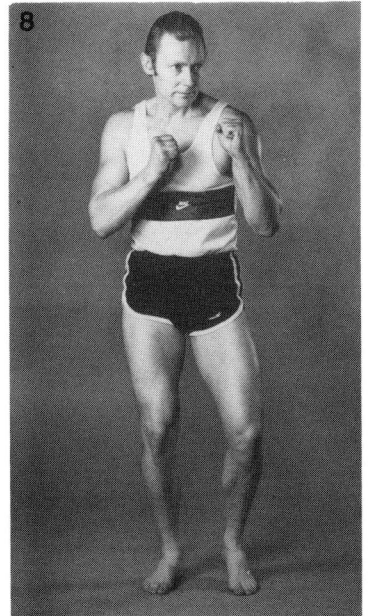

7 *Kick back-kick with the right leg.*

8 *Bring the kick back. Repeat the routine starting with a left roundhouse.*

Routine Six
Incorporating straight punch, and spinning crescent kick

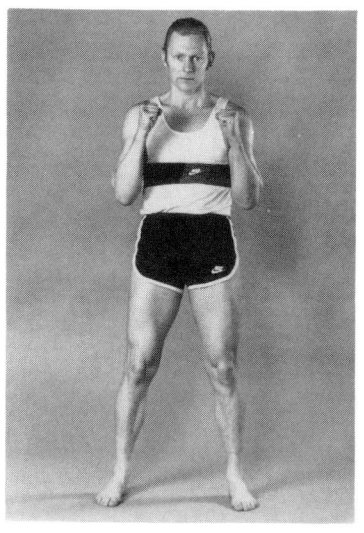

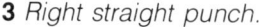

1 *Adopt ready position.*   **2** *Left straight punch.*

3 *Right straight punch.*   **4** *Left straight punch.*

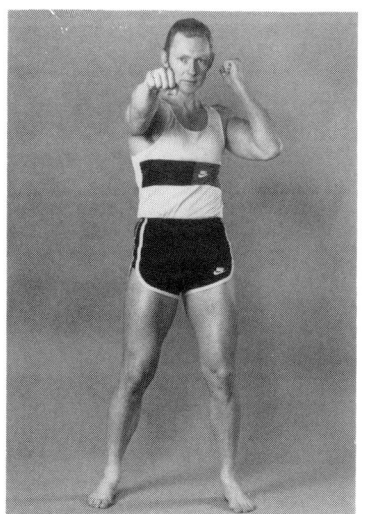

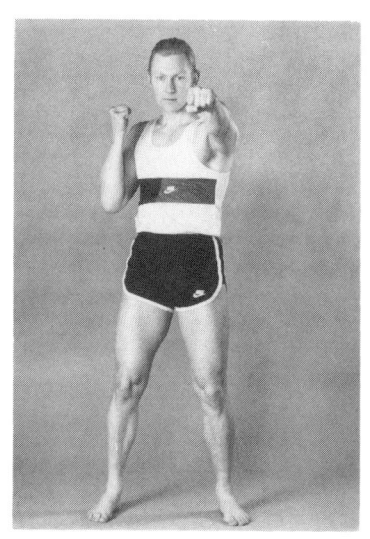

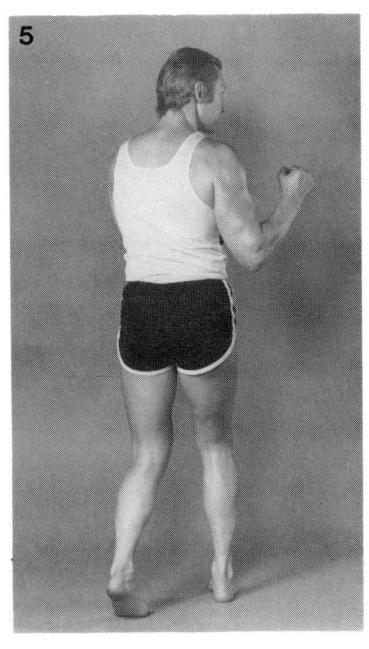

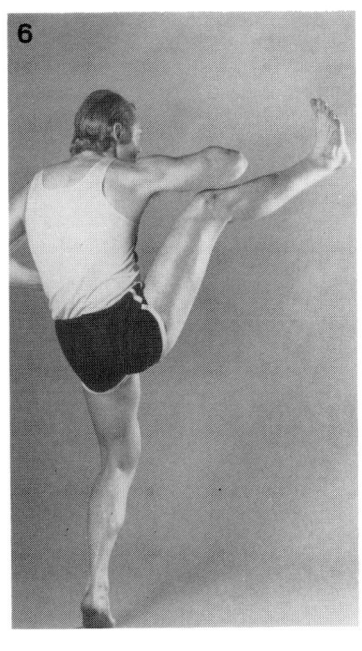

5 Spin to your right.

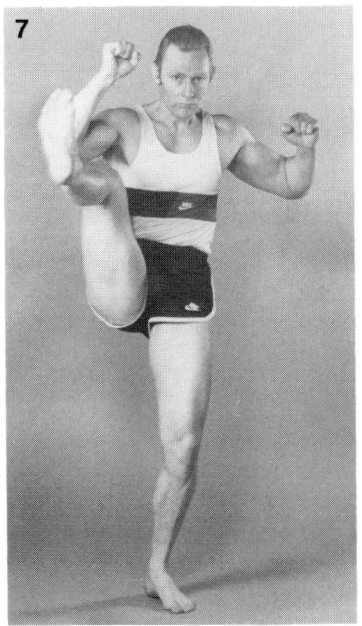

6 Start the spinning crescent kick two-thirds of the way round. You are kicking with your right leg.

7 Complete the spin, throwing the foot past your own face.

8 *Complete the kick.*

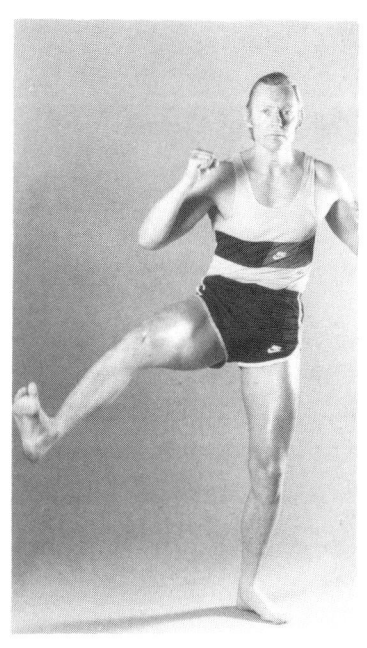

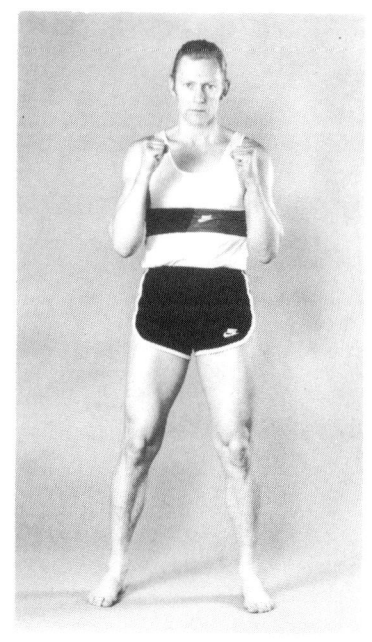

9 *Return to starting position. Begin again with a left straight punch. (This routine can also be performed the other way round beginning with a right straight punch).*

5
FREE DANCE

Routine One

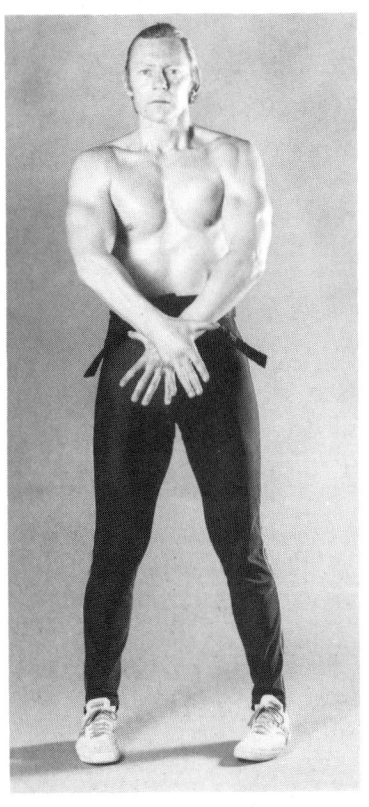

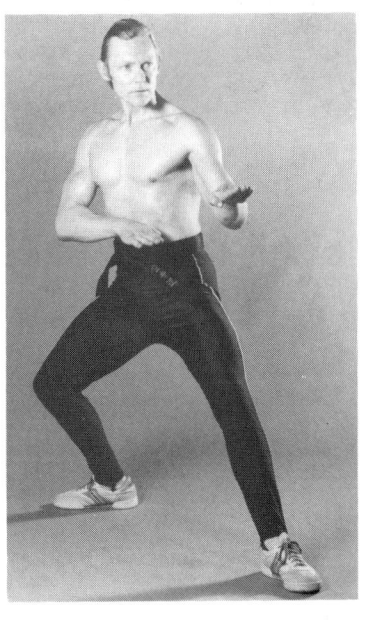

1 *Ready position. (All the following routines begin with this stance).*

2 *Step back with the right leg into back stance. About two-thirds of your bodyweight is on the back leg. The heels are in line and the feet at right-angles to each other. Both the hands are in a knifehand position with the palms facing downwards.*

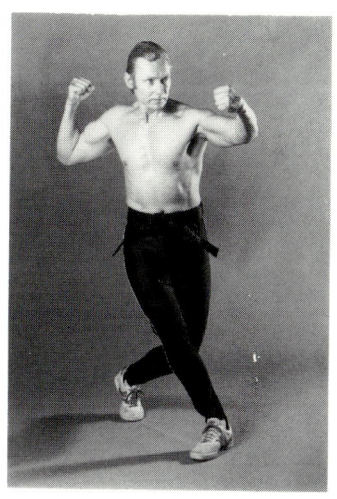

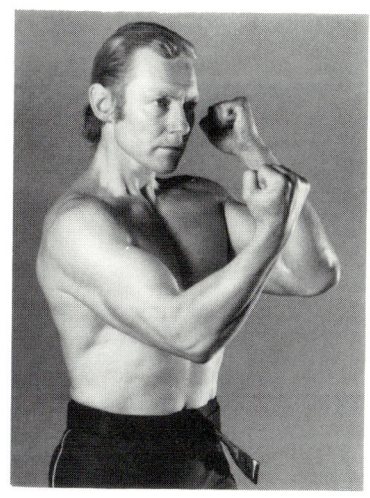

3 *Step forward with the right leg, turning the inside of the foot outwards. The left leg should be bent and the heel of the foot raised off the floor. Punch left hook as you step.*

4 *Step forward with the left leg and punch uppercut with the right fist as you step. This is the first punch of a multiple and should be performed speedily with the next two techniques.*

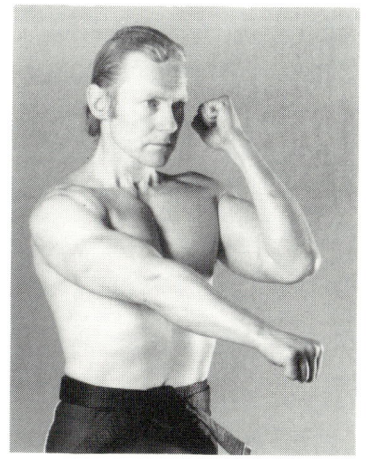

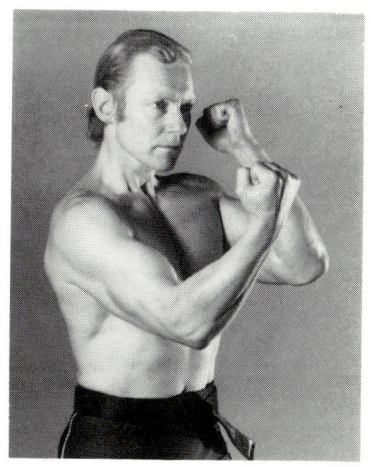

5 *Right straight punch.*

6 *Finish with another right uppercut.*

Routine Two

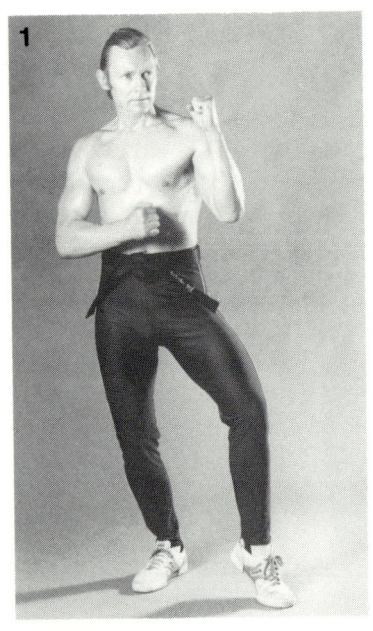

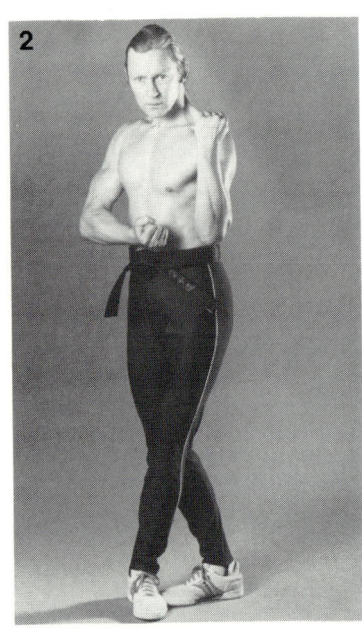

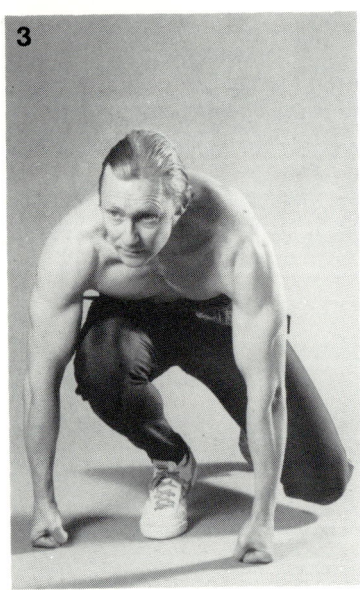

1 *Step back from ready position into cat stance. In this stance most of the weight is on the back leg which is bent. The foot of the back leg is turned at 45'. The front leg is also bent and rests on the ball of the foot. The hands make fists, one across the abdomen and the other raised in a guard.*

2 *Step forward with the left leg into T-stance with the feet intersecting at right angles.*

3 *Drop into a squat position on your right leg and punch the floor lightly with your fists.*

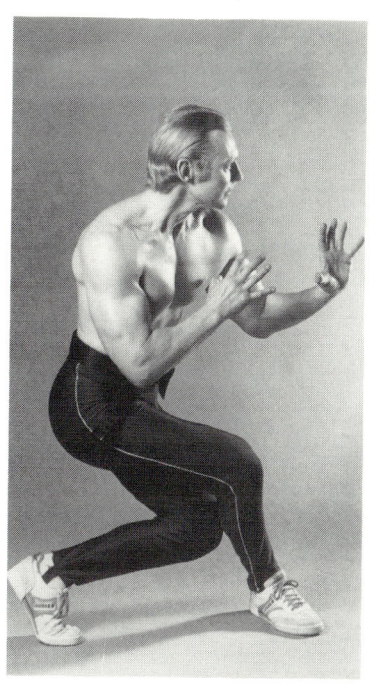

4 *Turn to your left, moving your right leg across and forward and rising slightly in the process. The fingers of the hands should be spread. Bend your left leg keeping the heel off the floor and tucking the knee in behind the knee of the right leg.*

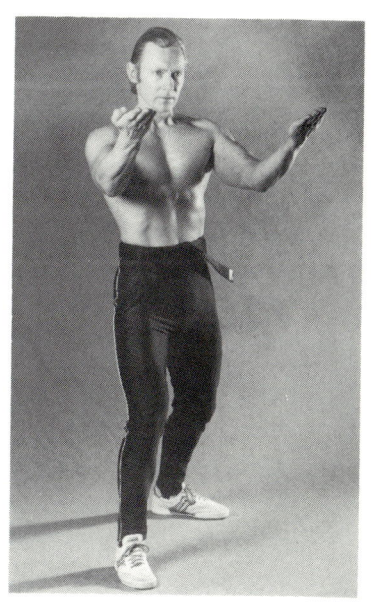

5 *Rise up and step with your right leg to face in the original direction. Make a knifehand shape with the hands as you step and make sure the palms are facing upwards.*

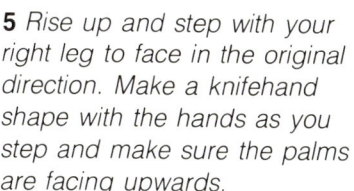

Routine Three

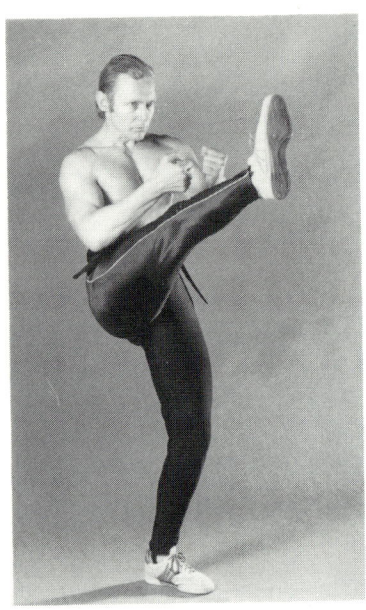

1 *From the ready position kick front-kick with the right leg.*

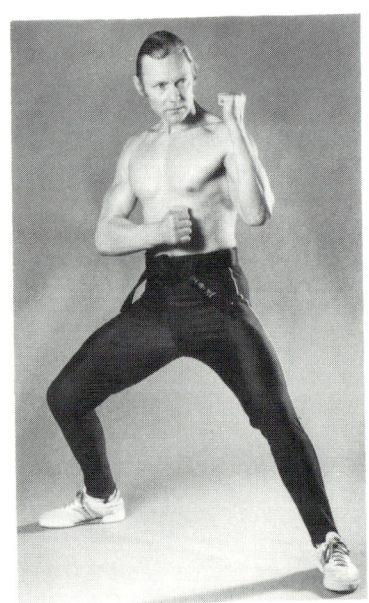

2 *Step straight back into back stance from the kick in a smooth uninterrupted motion.*

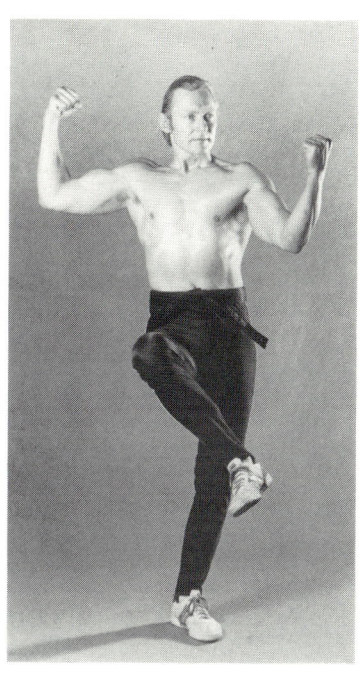

3 *Stand up on your left leg with your right crossed over the knee. Arms are in a tensed double-biceps posture.*

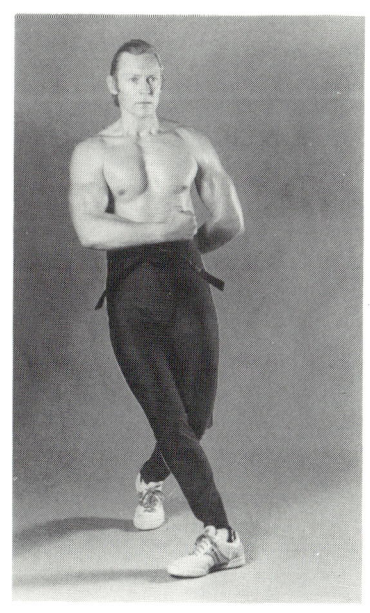

4 *Thrust your right leg forward and turn your foot so that the inside faces outwards. The left leg is bent and the heel is off the floor, while the knee is pressed against the back of the right knee. The right arm is flexed across the abdominals and the left arm is hooked round the back.*

Routine Four

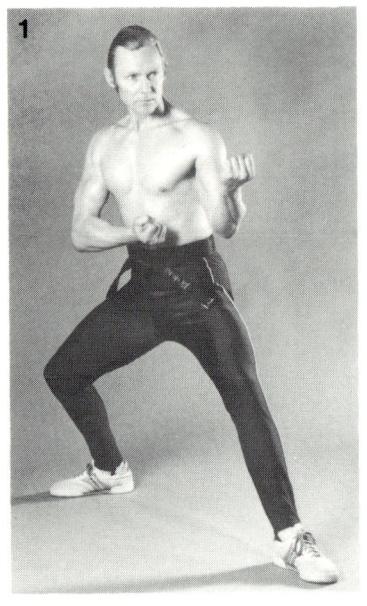

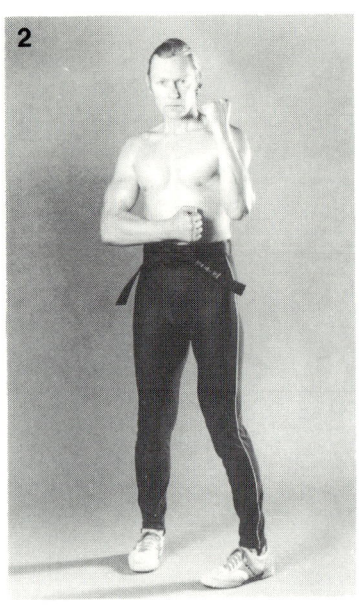

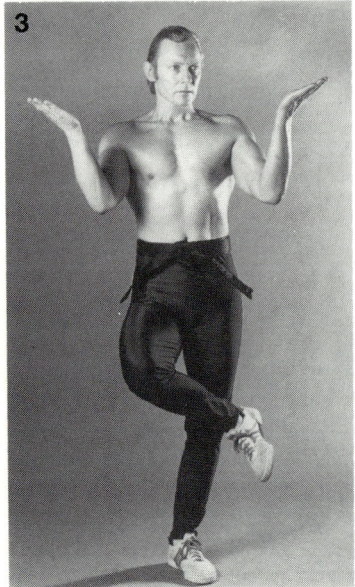

1 *Step back with the right leg from the ready stance into a back stance. Turn the fists upwards.*

2 *The base of the front foot then turns inwards and the back (right) leg pulls up towards the left into hourglass stance. The right foot points forwards and the knees are slightly bent inwards. The left fist is raised.*

3 *Bend your right leg across the knee of your left and turn to the right; open your hands into knifehand shape, palms facing up.*

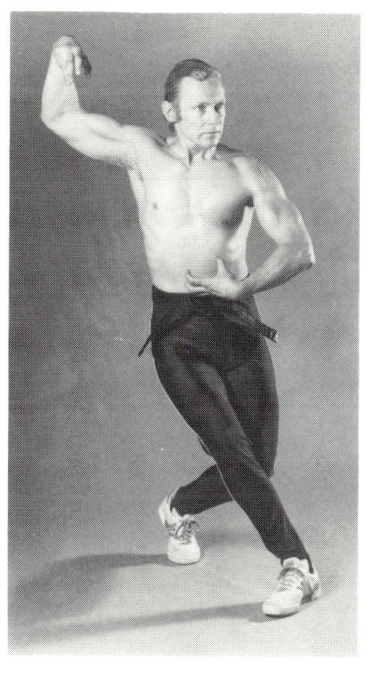

4 *The right leg now steps forward and straightens. The foot is turned with the inside facing out. The left leg is bent and the heel raised off the floor. The hands make claw shapes, the right raised to eye level or above and the left turned towards the stomach. The left knee presses into the back of the right.*

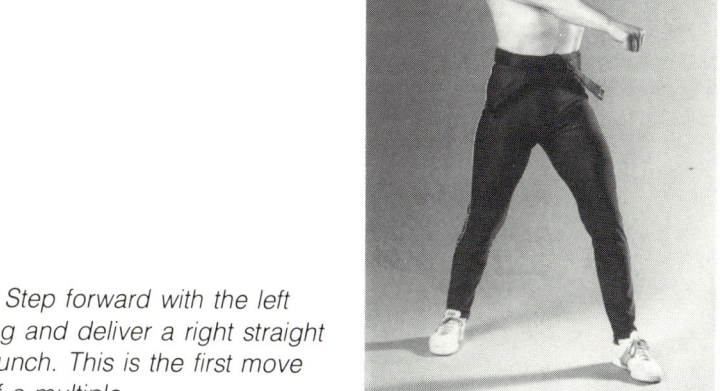

5 *Step forward with the left leg and deliver a right straight punch. This is the first move of a multiple.*

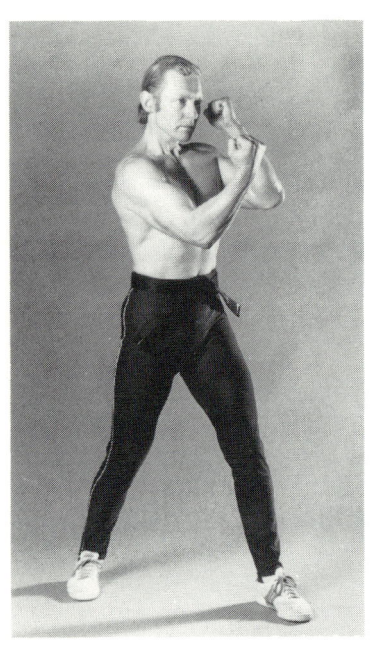

6 *With the same hand perform an uppercut.*

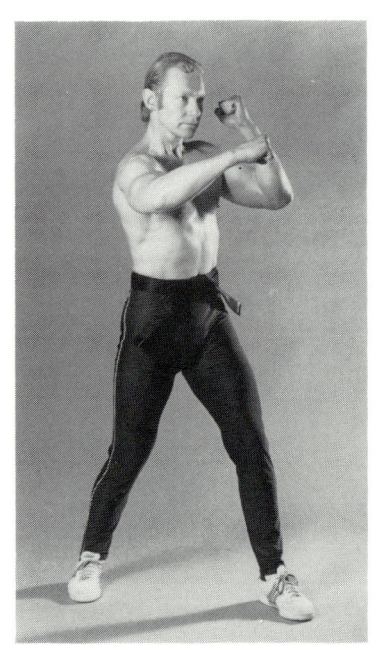

7 *Finish with a right hook.*

Routine Five

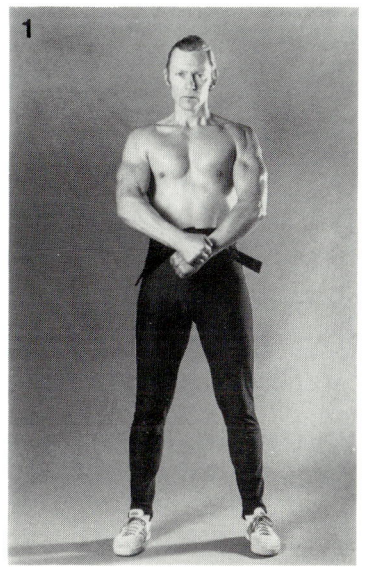

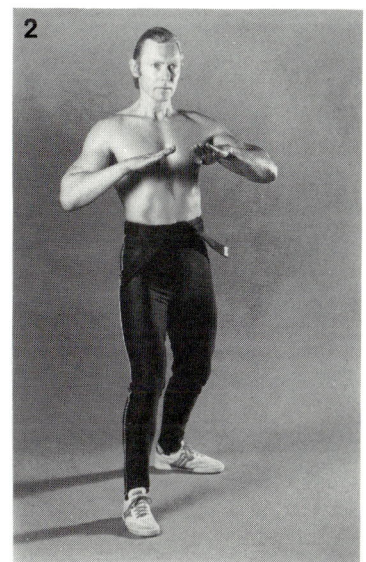

1 *Variation on ready posture — fists crossed.*

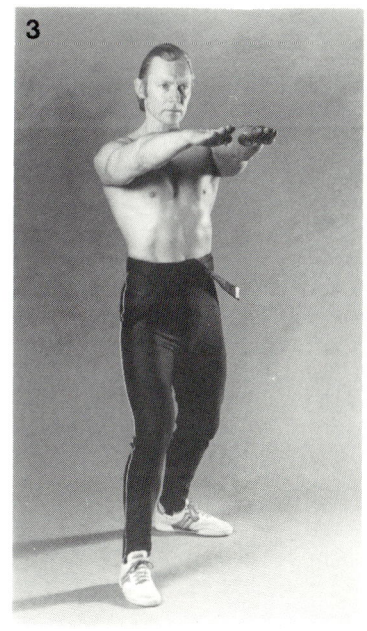

2 *While stepping forward with the right leg bring your hands up to your chest in knifehand position with the palms facing down.*

3 *Thrust hands forward in a spearhand strike.*

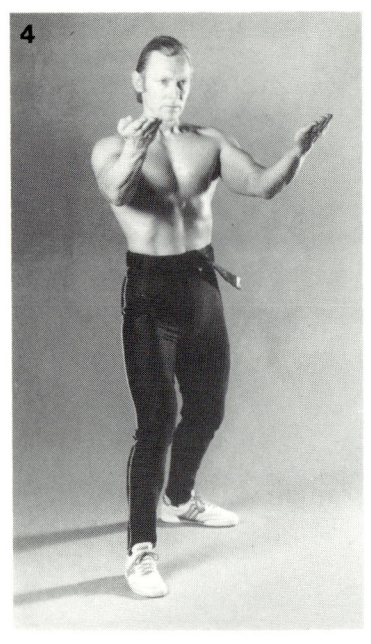

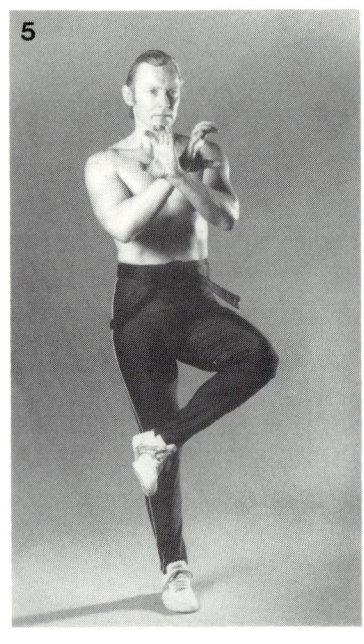

4 *Flip your hands over and perform double ridgehand strike.*

5 *Balance on your right leg. Bring your left leg across your right knee and cross your hands in a claw shape.*

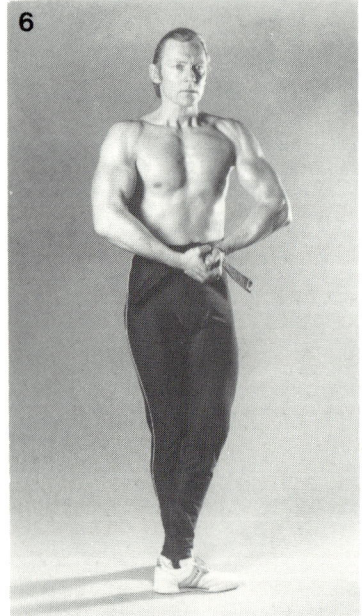

6 *Step down with your left foot into T-stance. Tense the muscles of the arms and torso by making a fist with your right hand and pushing it against the resistance of your left hand.*

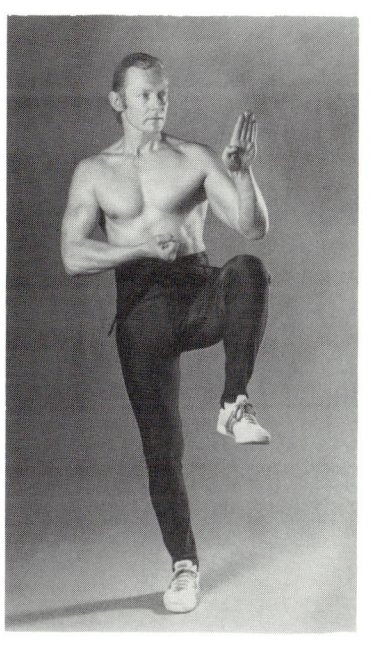

7 *Stand on your right leg and lift the left knee. Make a fist with your right hand and position it over your stomach. Make a knifehand shape with your left and turn the palm to face outwards.*

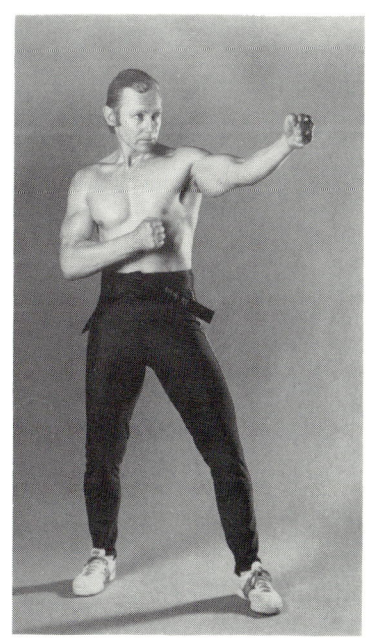

8 *Step down with the left leg and punch with a left jab. This is the first move of a multiple.*

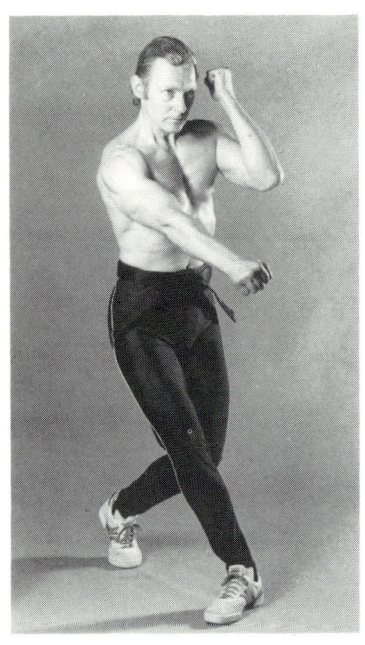

9 *Punch a straight punch with the right hand while stepping forwards with the right leg. Keep the heel of the left foot off the floor and turn out the right foot.*

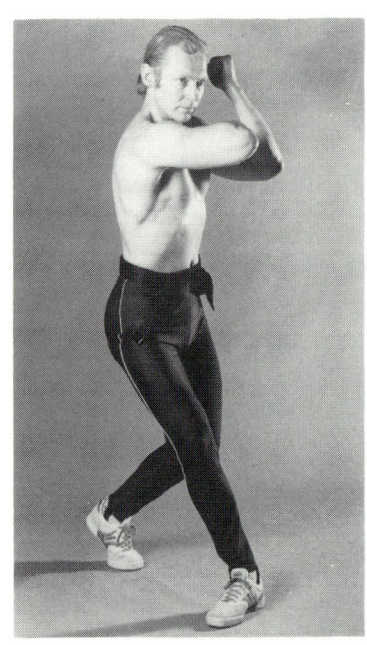

10 *Perform a right elbow strike.*

Multiples

These multiples can be performed in time to the beat or alternatively as fast hand movements that transcend the music. They should be practised until they can be performed with speed and without thinking.

Multiple One

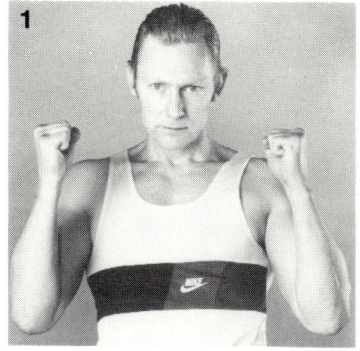

1 *Ready stance.*

2 *Bring your right fist back to your hip.*

3 *Punch uppercut.*

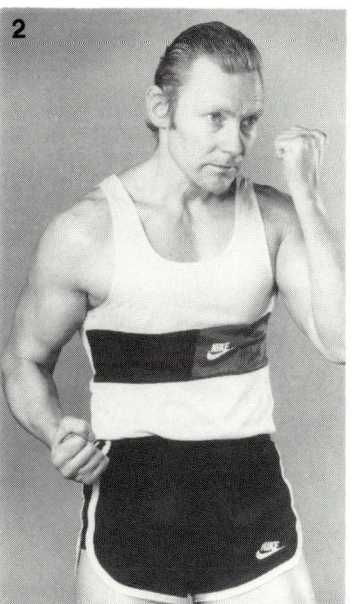

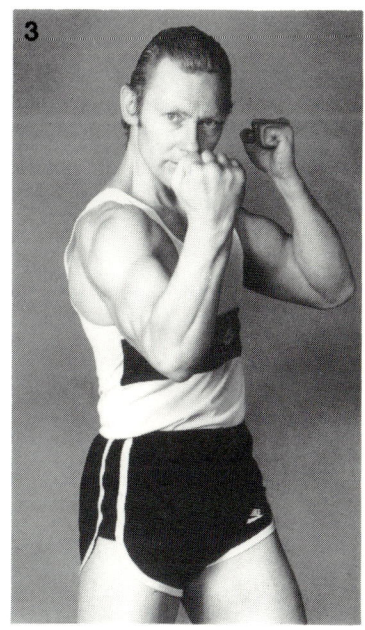

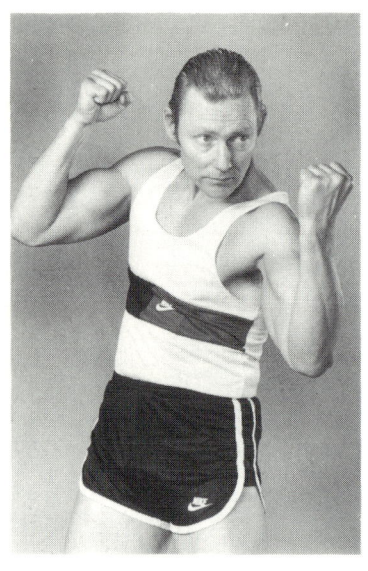

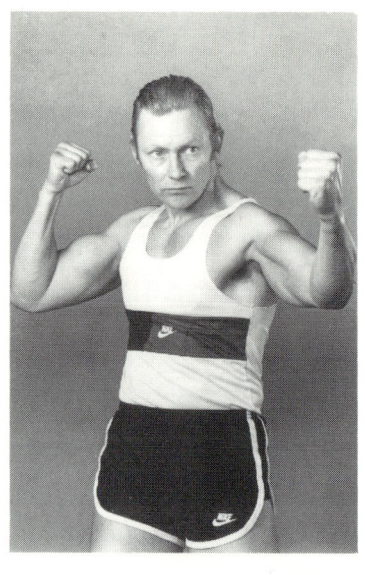

4 *Punch left uppercut.*

5 *Punch left hook.*

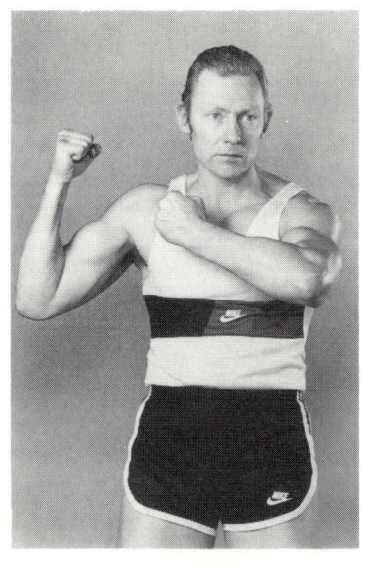

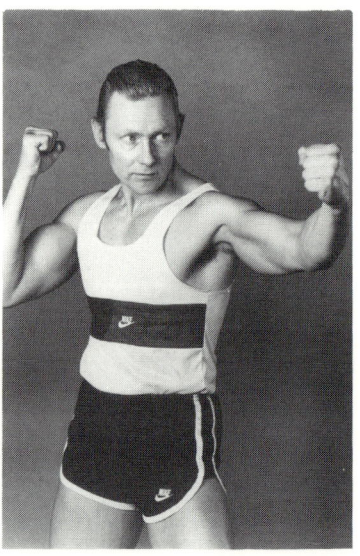

6 *Bring your left fist back to your right shoulder.*

7 *Strike backfist.*

Multiple Two

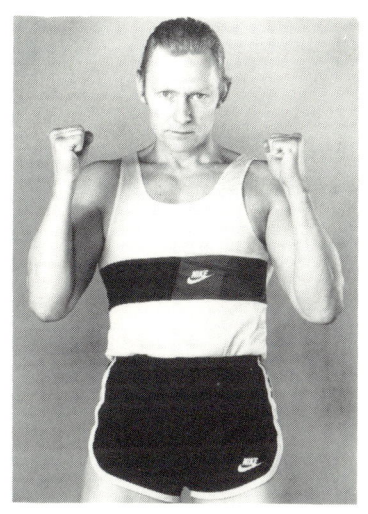

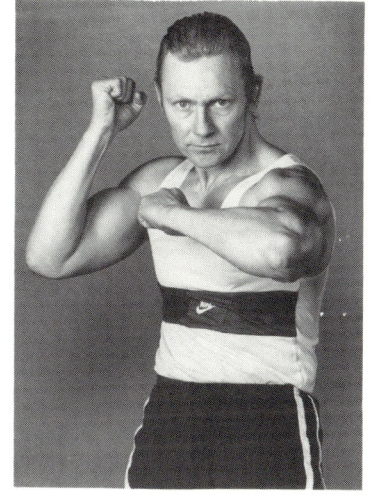

1 *Ready position*

2 *Left elbow strike (inward).*

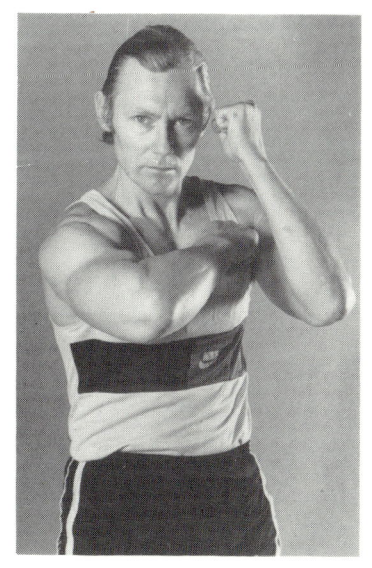

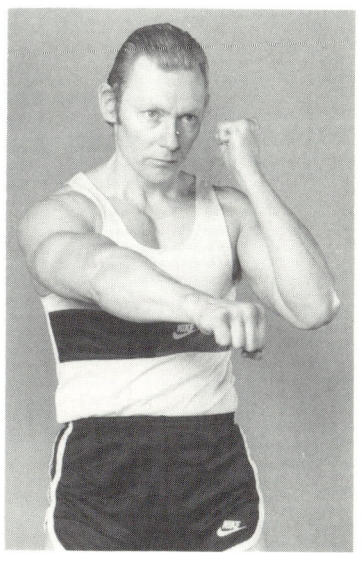

3 *Right elbow strike (inward).*

4 *Right straight punch.*

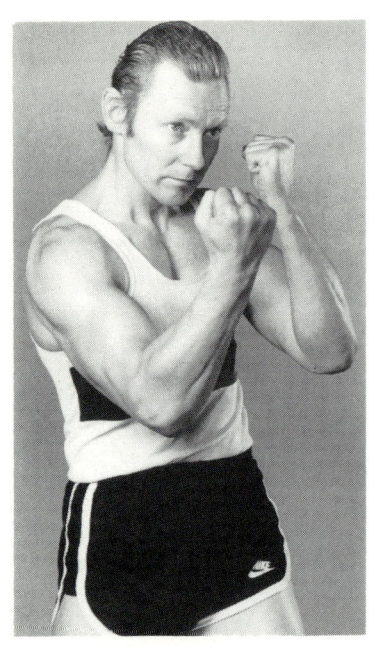

5 *Right uppercut.*

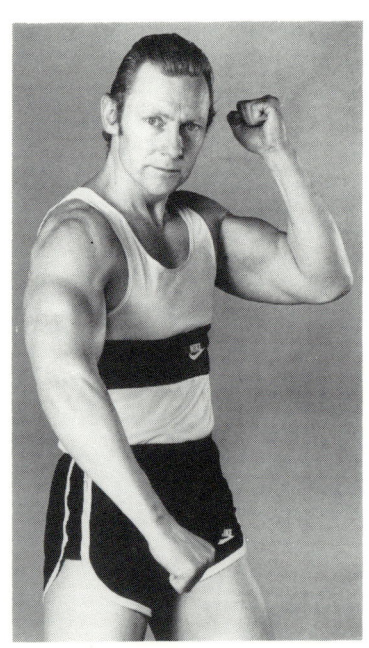

6 *Right hammerfist (to the groin area).*

6

POSTURES

In the martial arts most of the stances have names, although different styles may sometimes have different names for the same stances. Nomenclature is not important or even practical in martial dance. The basic stances are named but as martial dance is infinitely creative and experimental, postures and stances proliferate. In their translation from bodybuilding and budo to martial dance these postures become modified as they are worked into the new mould and adapted to individual personalities and different body types. Whereas in the traditional martial arts the body is made to fit the kata and must subscribe to draconian rules of technique, in martial dance the movements and postures are not rigidly laid down as laws but are intended as a basis from which to develop stylistic individuality. Everyone's body or morphology is different, everyone's personality unique, and therefore it is logical that each dancer must find his or her own way of moving and interpreting the standard units.

Like a cell dividing, a posture can give rise to permutations of itself. An on-going creative process can be sparked off that spawns postures in never-ending abundance, yet all of them are off-shoots from the same family, manifesting the soul of their original source — the essential flavour of martial arts locomotion.

Martial dance is really a showcase for the endless configurations of the human body. It is a statement invoking our awareness of how many different ways there are in which a dancer can arrange his or her body to create an exciting bodyline. Postures become almost an art within an art.

Dancing entails a progressively enriched awareness of and empathy with the body's ability to set itself in multiple configurations and to move smoothly and rhythmically from one to another. This is a subtle concept. It is not easy to appreciate the body at this level for too many of us take our bodies for granted and do not fully realize this distinctly human genius. No animal is remotely equal to us or our ability to use our bodies creatively in spacial compositions of poetic stance.

The following postures are an introduction to the art of rhythmic posing. Practise them one by one and then begin to experiment with them, making up your own combinations and putting them to music. Limit yourself to four or five postures in each sequence, and when you feel happy and confident with these try fusing them with multiples and on-the-spot routines — even the aerobic exercises.

Moving To Music

The free dance routines and the postures illustrated in this book can be performed to many types of music and many tempos. To start with choose a moderately slow pop record and fit a count of one...two...three...four...to the rhythm. Then try hitting a different posture to each count. When you get used to moving in this way to the count you will gradually be able to move instinctively and automatically and to dispense with counting altogether.

You are an individual so discover your own way of moving and expressing these postures. There are really no rules as long as all your movements have integrity. Here are a few suggested combinations using the postures:

1   1-7-21-23
2   32-8-10-24
3   12-15-3-35
4   19-13-22-34
5   36-18-27-30

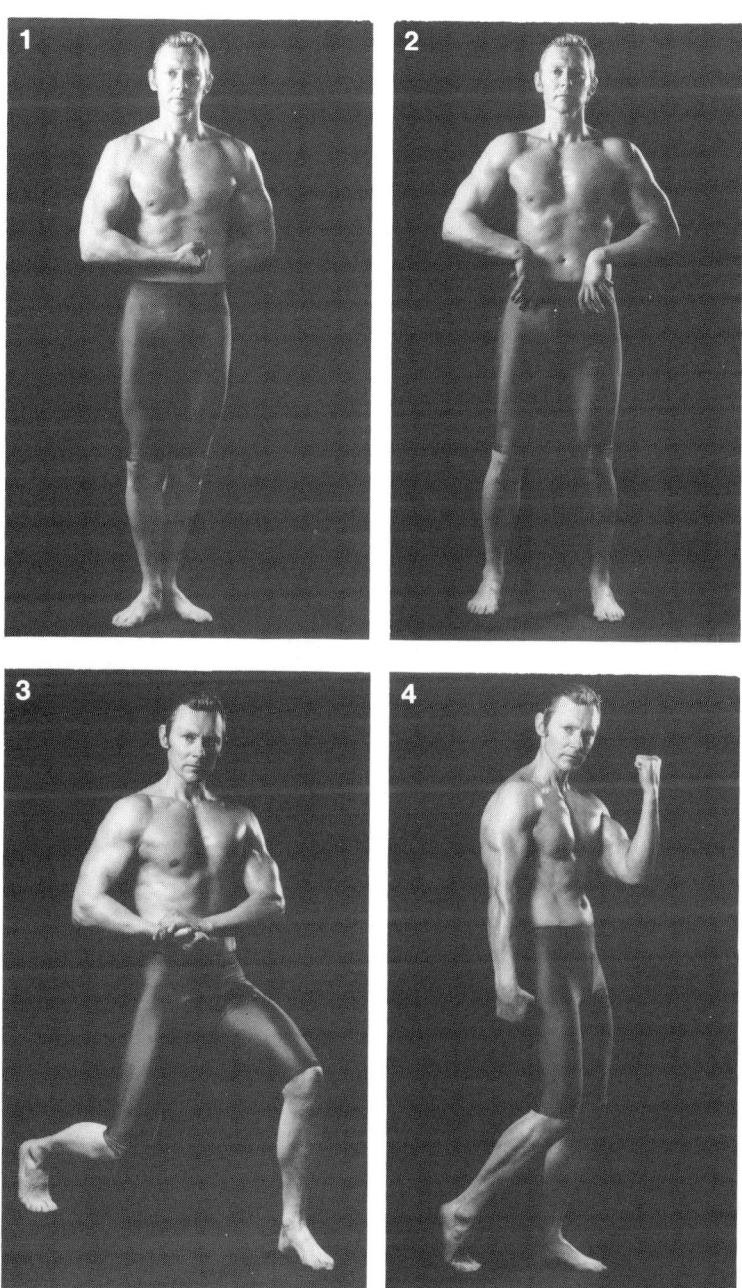

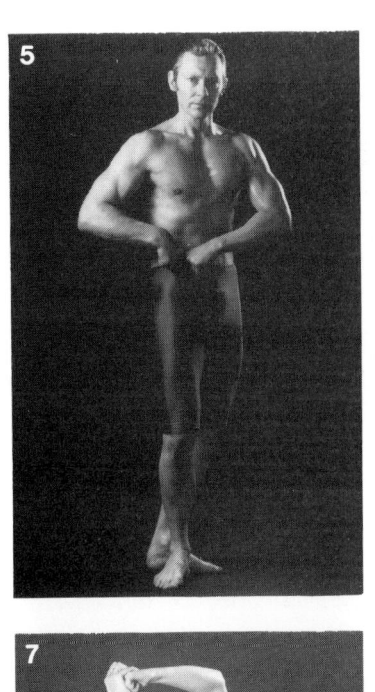

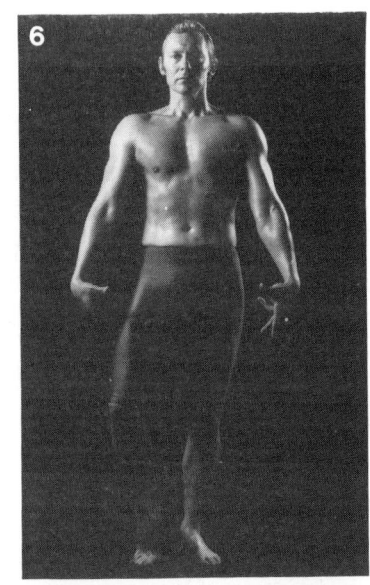

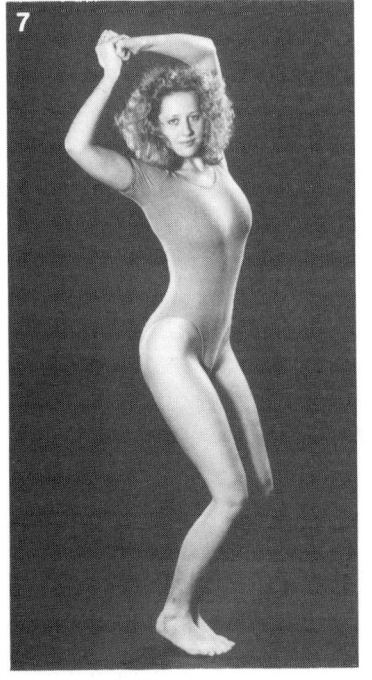

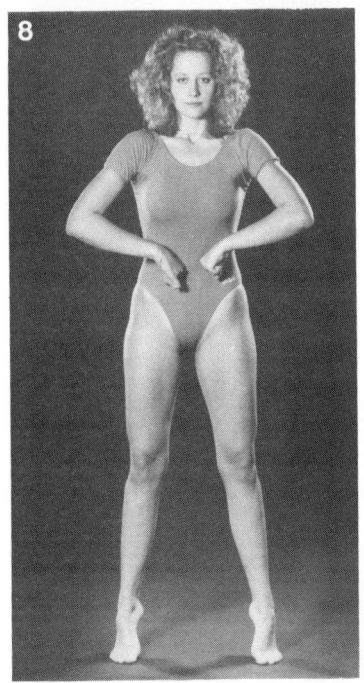

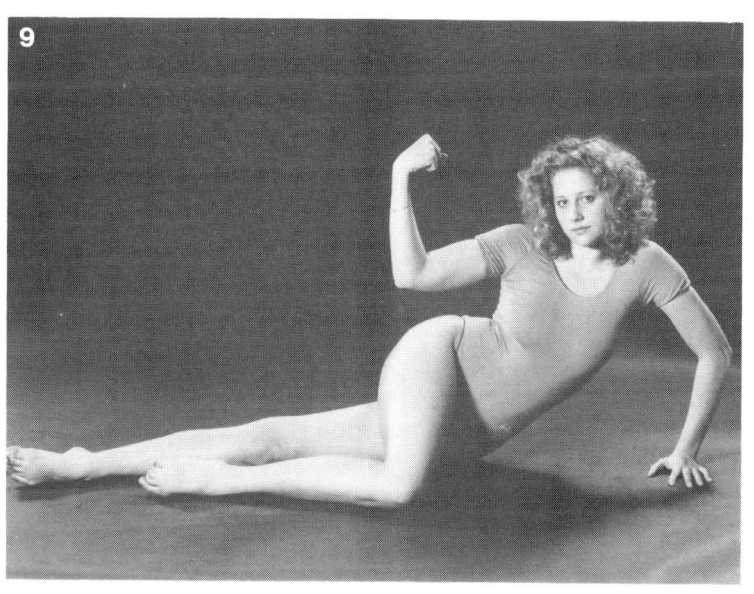

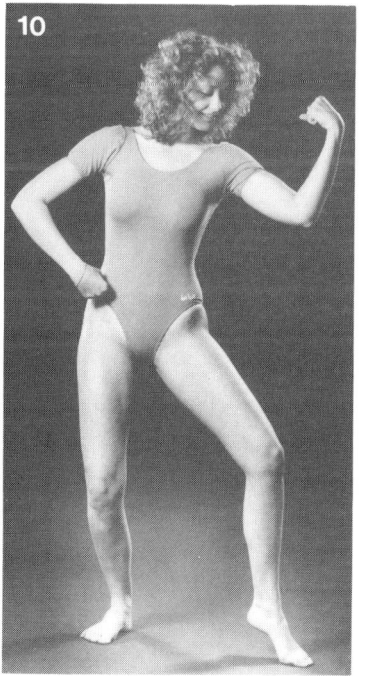

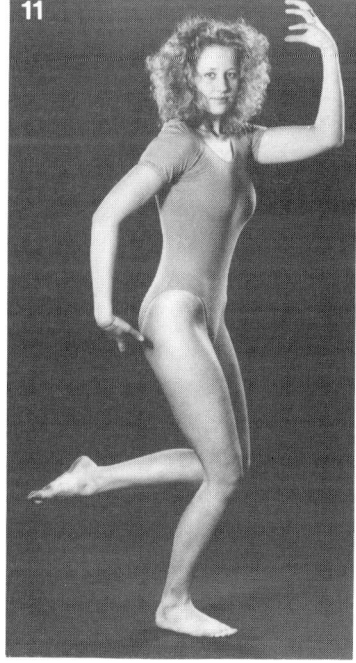

149

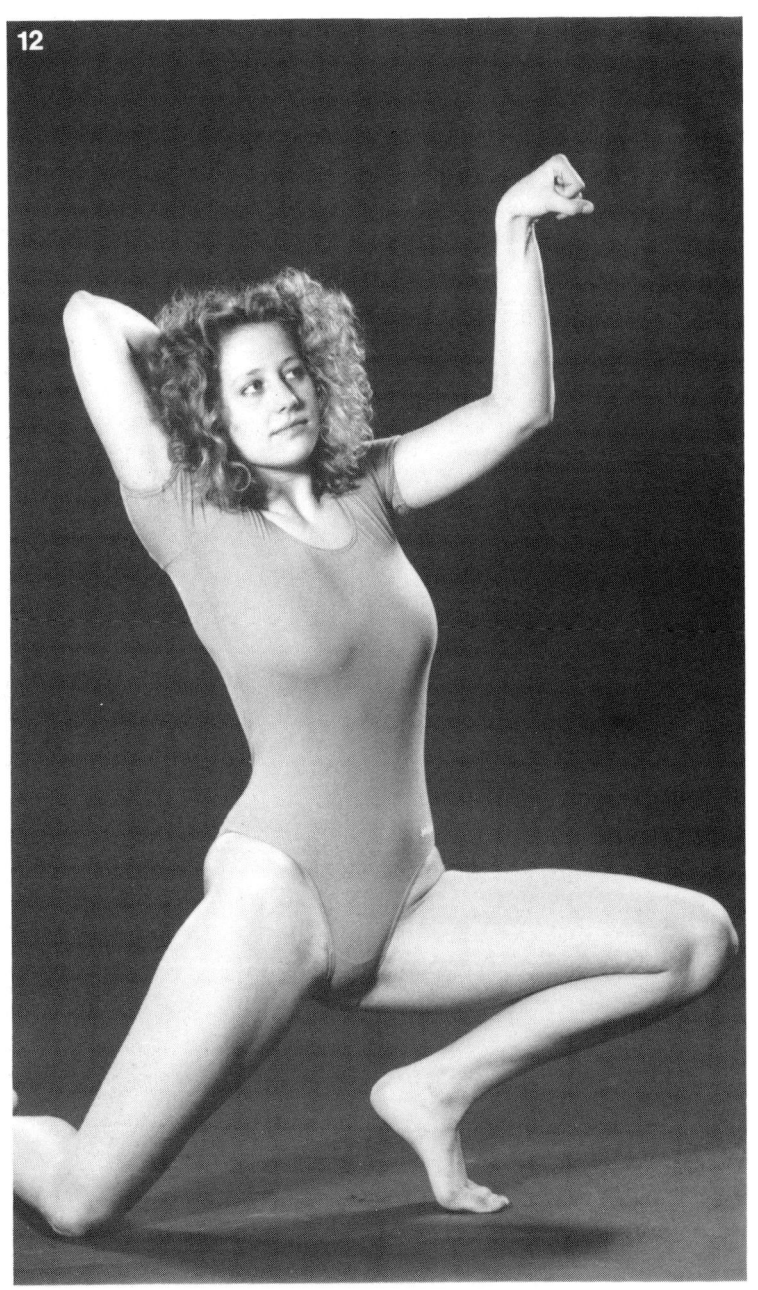

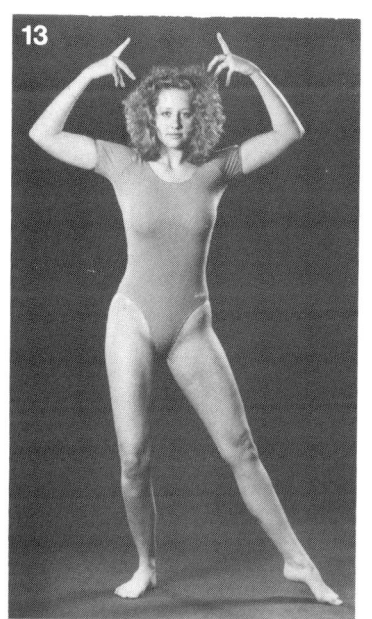

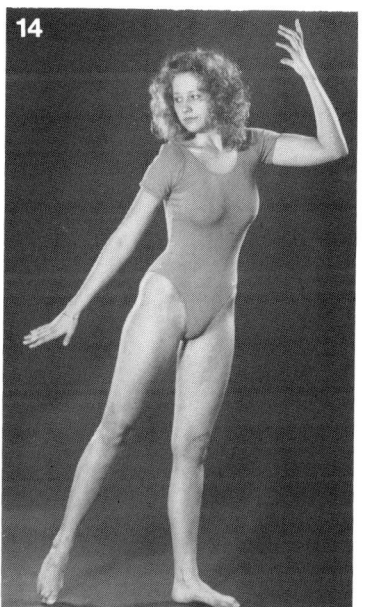

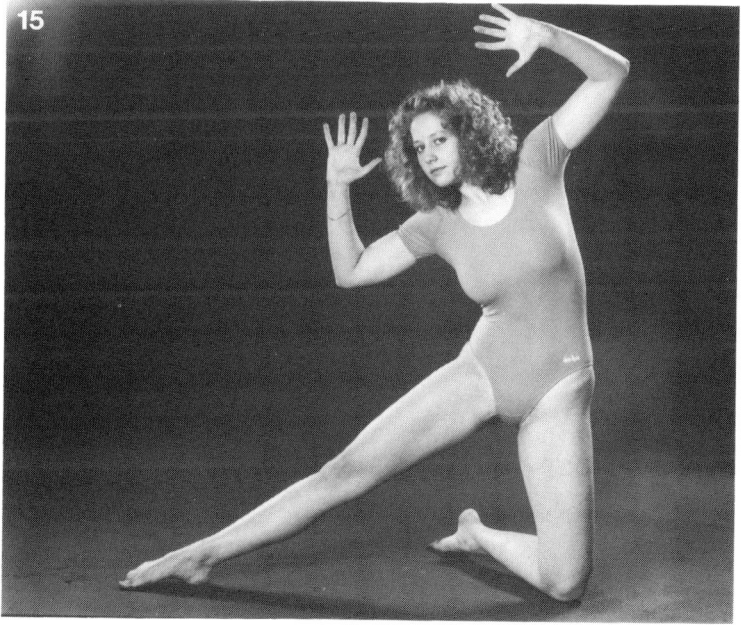

151

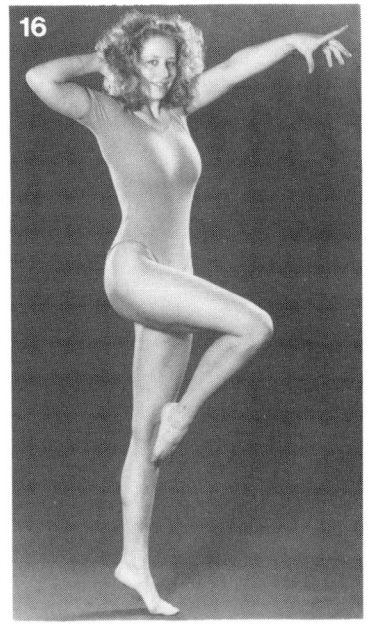
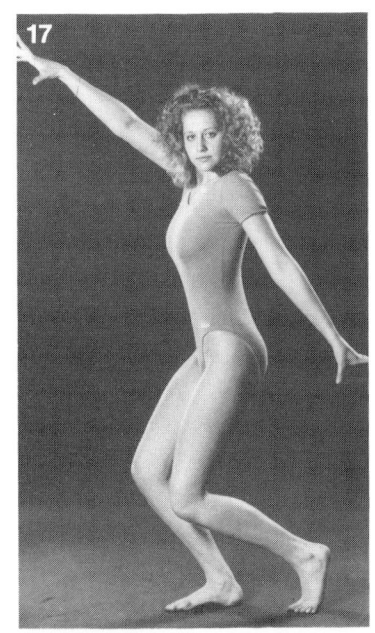
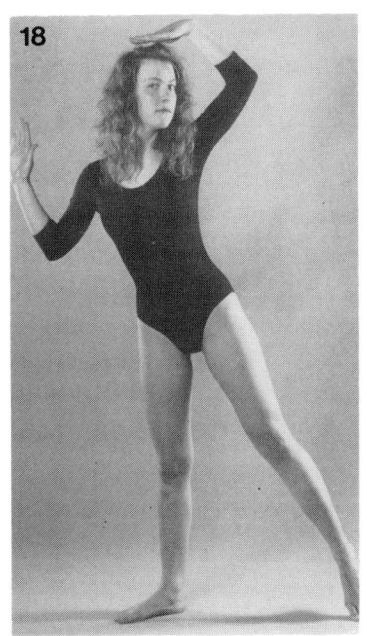
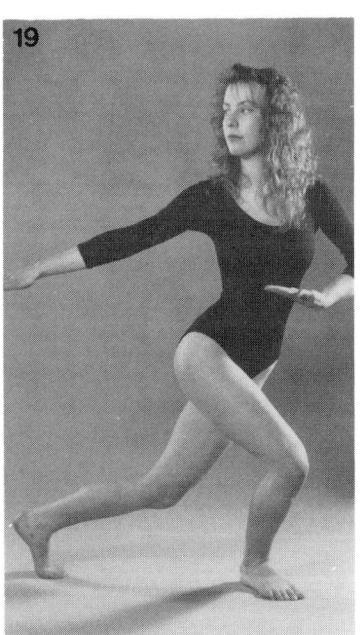

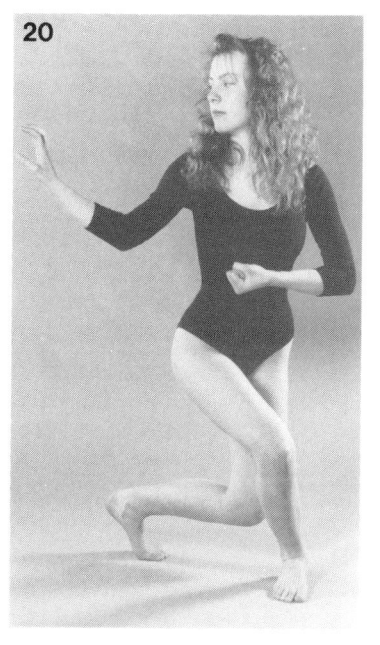
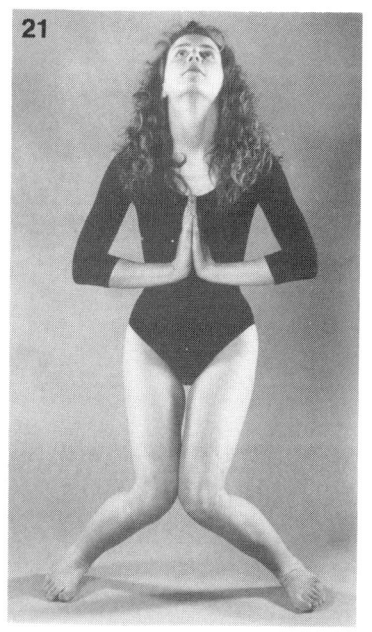

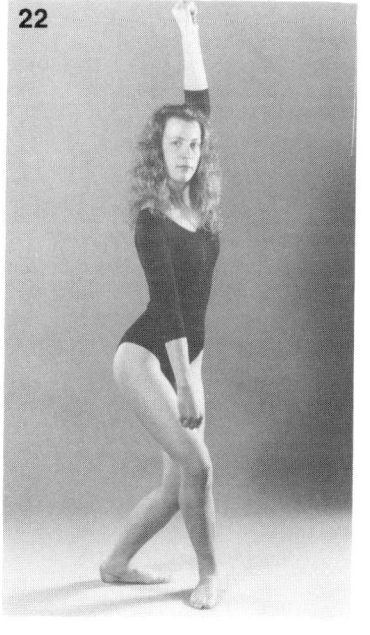
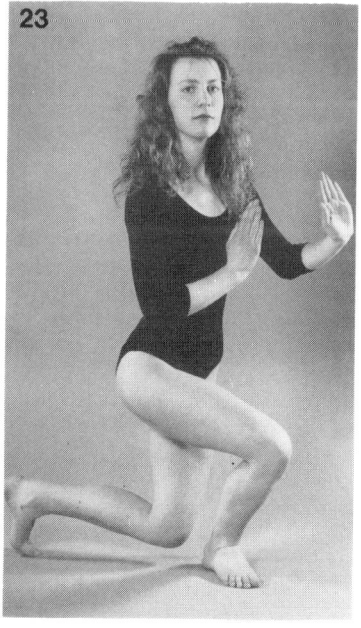

153

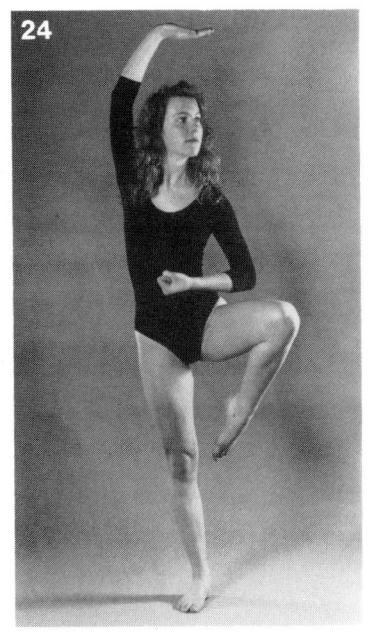

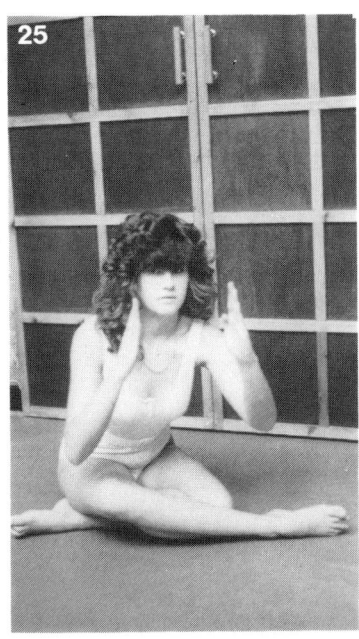

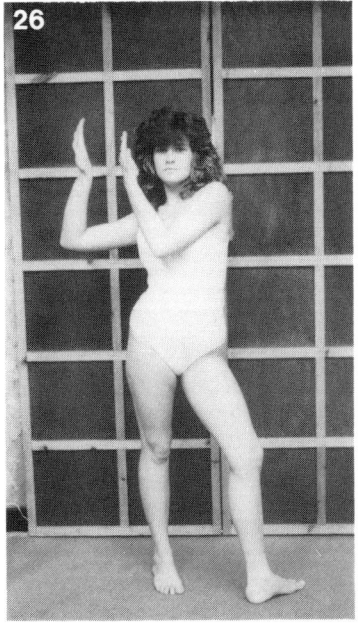

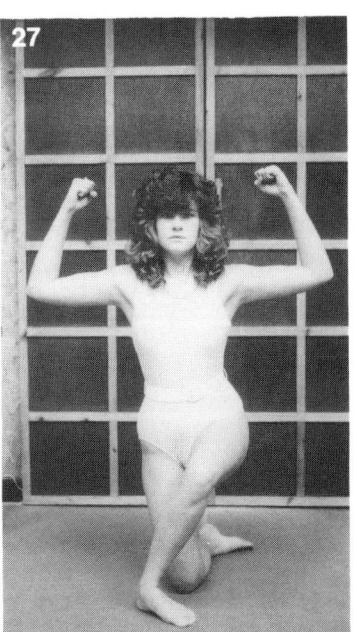

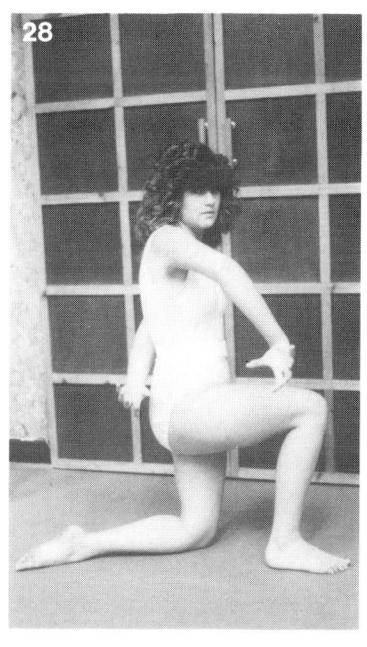
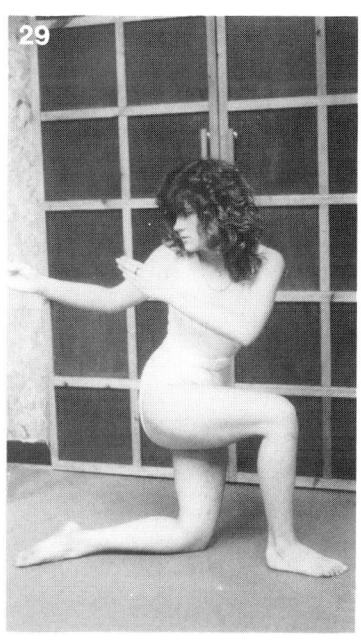
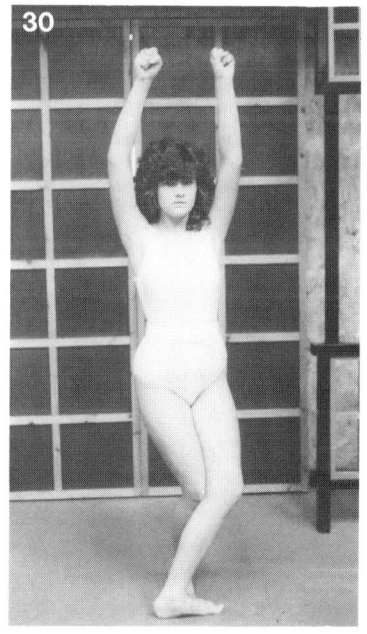
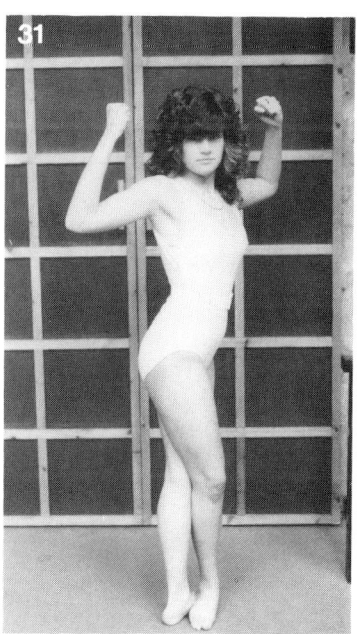

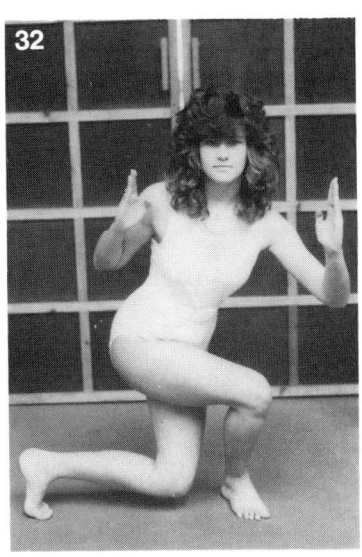

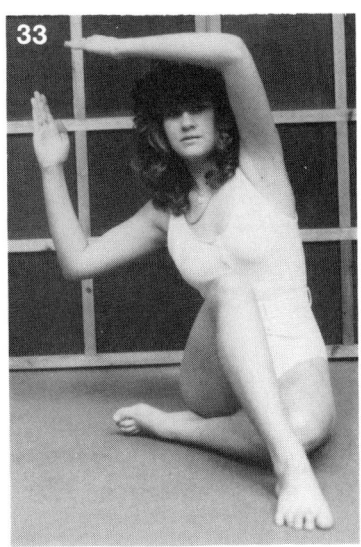

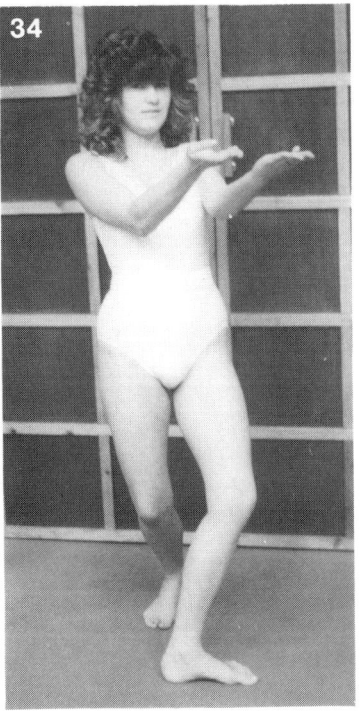

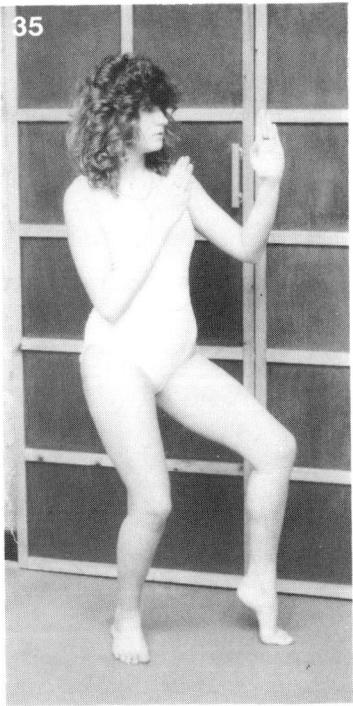

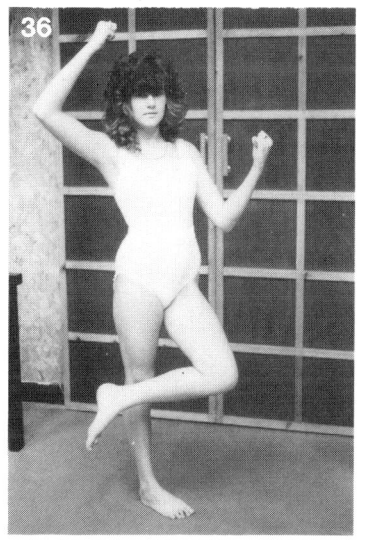
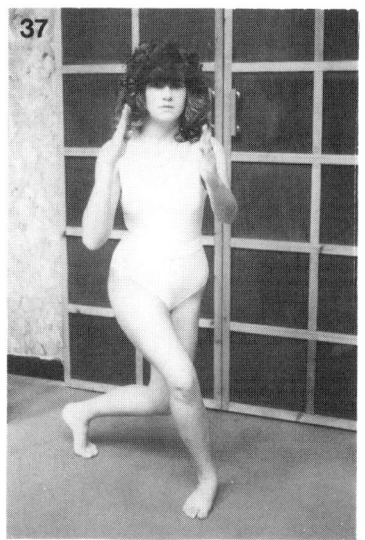
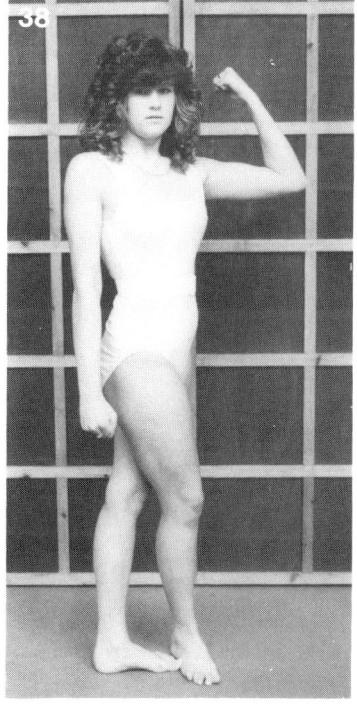
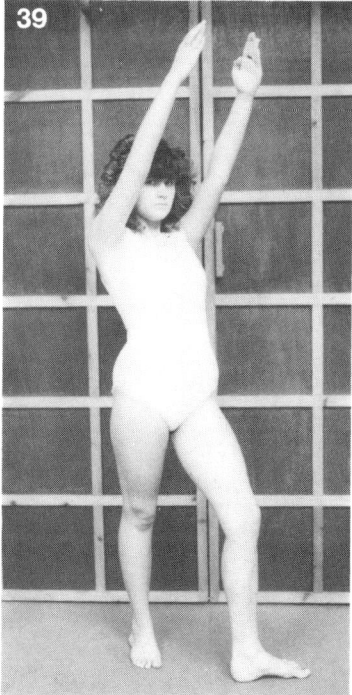

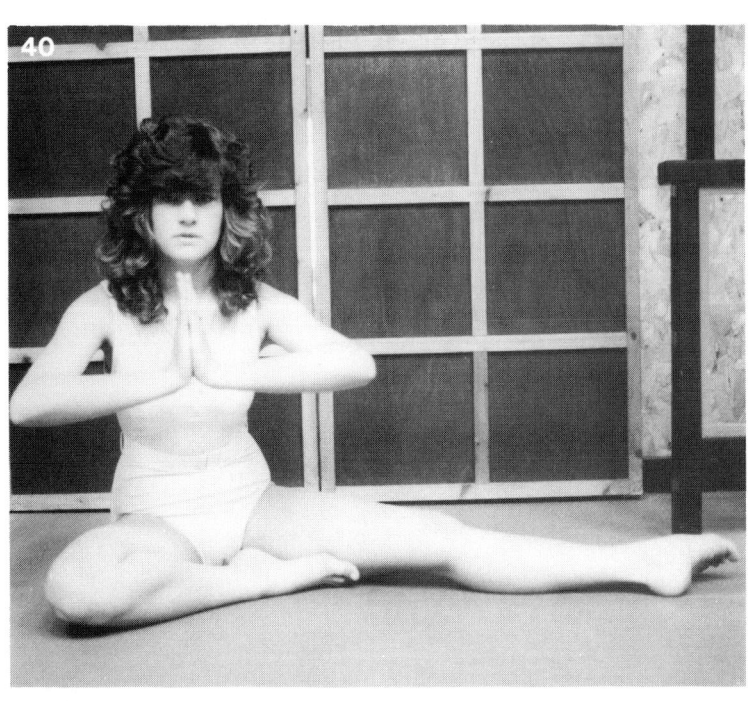

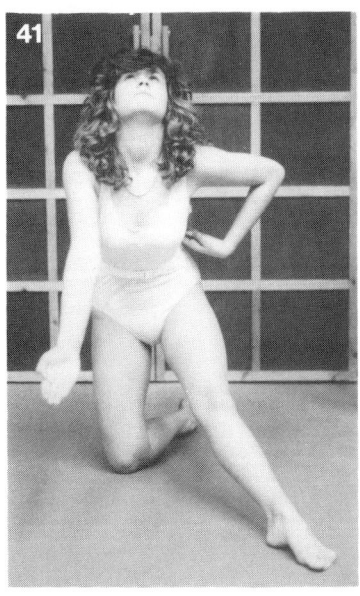

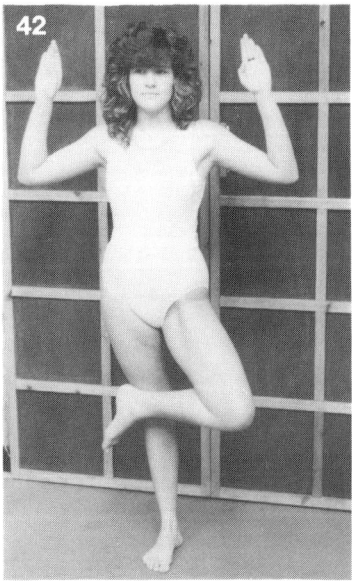

APPENDIX
WEIGHT TRAINING—
GYMWORK

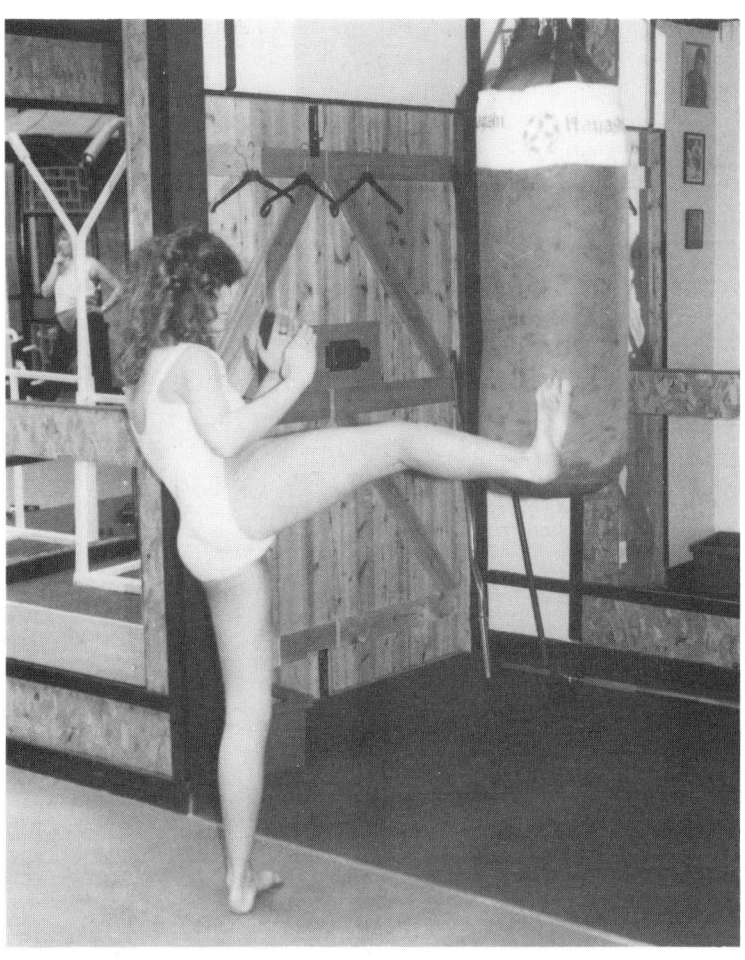

Working from the principle of choosing one exercise for each part of the body, the training programme that follows is a complete body workout that should ideally be performed three times a week with a day for recovery between each. The correct poundage will vary from person to person but should be heavy enough to fatigue the muscles at the end of each set. Each set should entail from eight to ten repetitions and one should do four to five sets of every exercise in the programme.

Exercises give the best results if they are performed

strictly without swinging the weight—breathing is also important. One should breathe out while actually performing the exercise and breathe in on the negatives. For example, if you are pressing a barbell above your head you should breathe out as you push it up and in as you lower it. The weight at all times should be controlled and the exercise carried out moderately slowly.

It is also important not to waste time chatting in the gym, especially in between sets for the same body-part. If you have to talk, do it between body-parts — for example, don't break off for a drawn-out chin-wag in the middle of doing your biceps or you will lose the 'pump'. Do all five sets of biceps curls in close sequence and then, if you have to, take a short break before going on to another body-part. The whole workout should be done as quickly as possible (without rushing) because you don't want to spend longer in the gym than you have to. There is no hard rule about how long to rest between sets but your work-rate should keep you slightly out of breath for the whole duration of the workout.

It is a good rule to begin your workout with squats. Always warm up with a very low poundage set, whatever body-part you are exercising. Aftermath muscle-soreness for the inexperienced will be an inconvenience until the body becomes acclimatized to the demands made upon it.

Variations

After the first programme has been tried for a few months there is a danger of slipping into a rut. You can get stale doing the same workout for too long. The more exercises you know, the greater is the opportunity to alternate them. For each body part there are several different exercises and by substituting one for another you will not only make your workouts more enjoyable but your results will be better and your gains faster. For example, you can give barbell curls a rest and try dumbell curls instead, or forego squats and use the leg machine. This way you are still exercising the same part of the body but with a different exercise.

Exercise One: Legs

Barbell Squats

It is best to do this exercise with the aid of a squat rack or stands, but while light weights are being used the barbell can be picked off the floor and placed on the back of the shoulders. Feet should be about shoulder-width apart. In a powerful exercise like the squat it is essential to remember the rules about breathing. Inhale deeply on the way down, exhale while coming up. To avoid the danger of losing your balance it is important to remember to keep your upper body upright and your head up so that you look straight in front of you at all times.

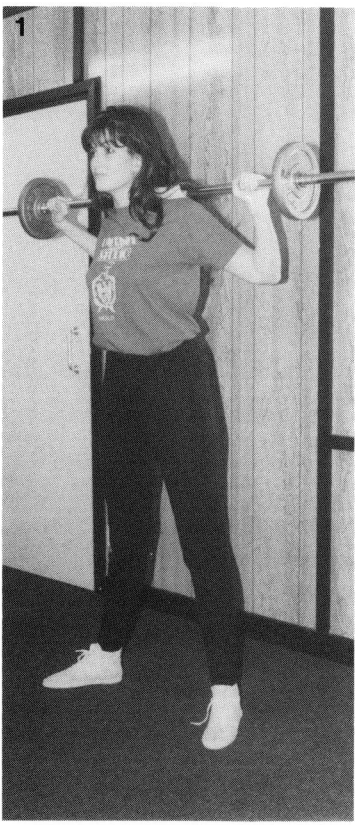

1 *Pick the bar up and place it on your back.*

2 *Squat, keeping your head up. Return to starting position and repeat.*

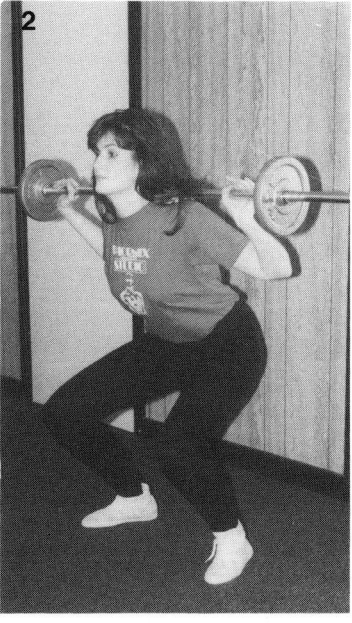

Variation: Dumbell Squats

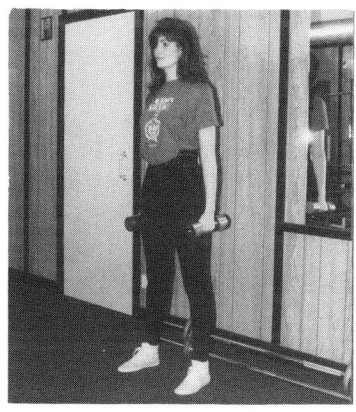 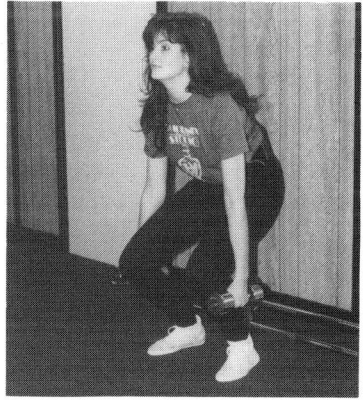

1 *Take a dumbell in each hand and stand with your feet shoulder-width apart.*

2 *Squat, keeping your head up. Return to starting position and repeat.*

Variation: Leg Extensions

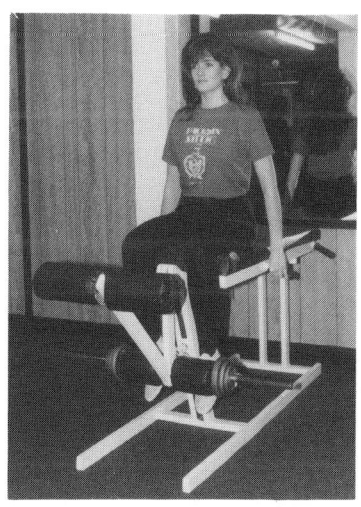 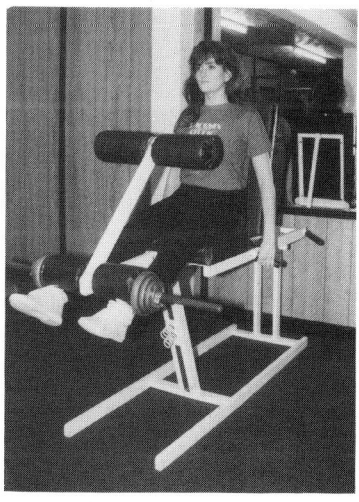

1 *Sit on the leg machine and hook your feet under the lower rollers.*

2 *Straighten your legs and return to the starting position slowly.*

Variation: Leg Curls

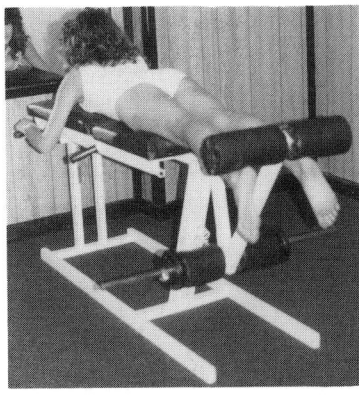 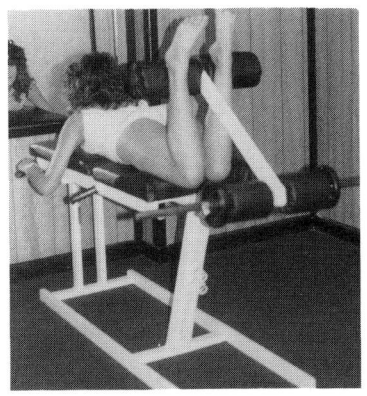

1 *Lie down on the leg machine and hook your heels under the top rollers.*

2 *Curl the weight as far as it will go and return to the starting position.*

Exercise Two: Chest

Bench Press

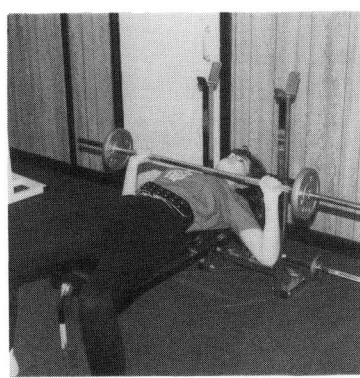 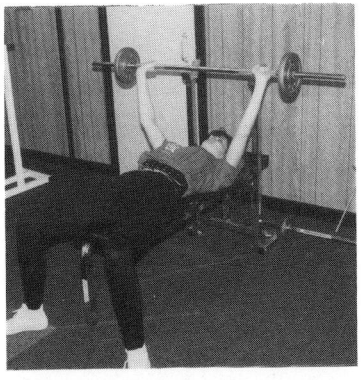

1 *Lie down on the exercise bench and using a fairly wide grip take the bar off the stand and lower it down to your upper chest.*

2 *Thrust the weight straight up and lock out your arms. Control the weight each time you lower it. The down movement should be relatively slow and the up movement a vigorous thrust.*

Variation: Flys

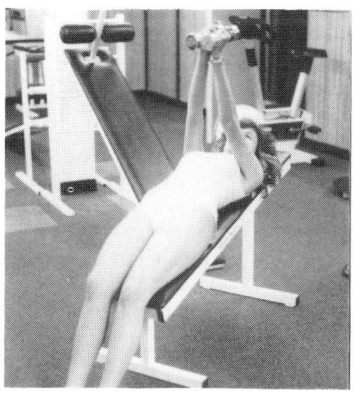 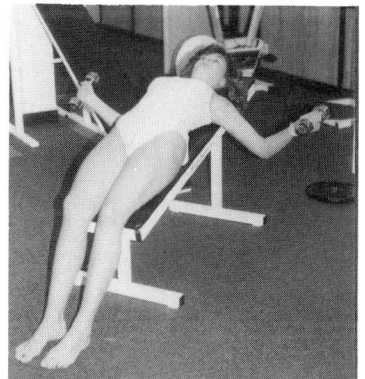

1 *Lie on the exercise bench (the bench may be flat or inclined). Hold the dumbells above you.*

2 *Lower the dumbells in a curved movement keeping the arms slightly bent at all times. If you are doing the exercise correctly you should feel a good stretching sensation in the shoulders and upper chest. Keeping your arms bent, return to position* **1**.

Variation: Pec-Deck

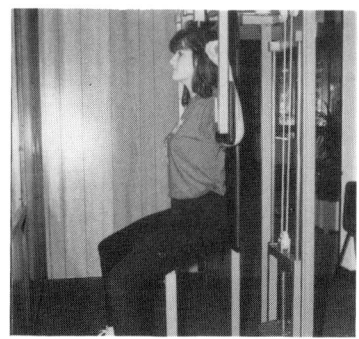 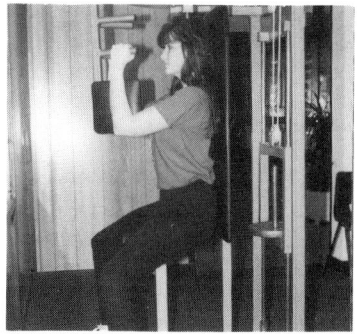

1 *Sit down on the seat provided and hook your arms round the arm rests.*

2 *Bring your forearms together to meet in front of you.*

Exercise Three: Shoulders (Deltoids)
Front Press

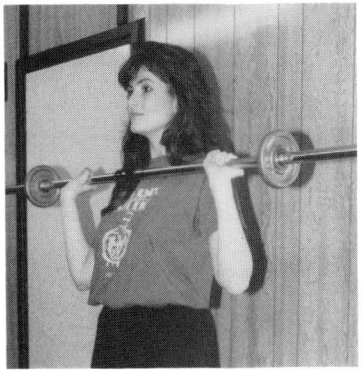 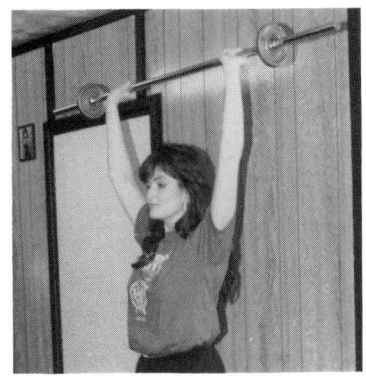

1 *Take a grip on the bar wider than your shoulders and lift it from the floor to your chest area.*

2 *Press it slowly over your head and lock your elbows. Lower it to your chest and press again.*

Variation: Behind Neck Press

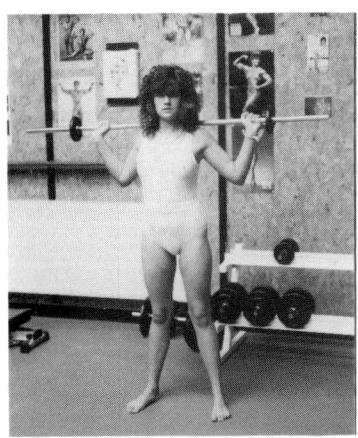 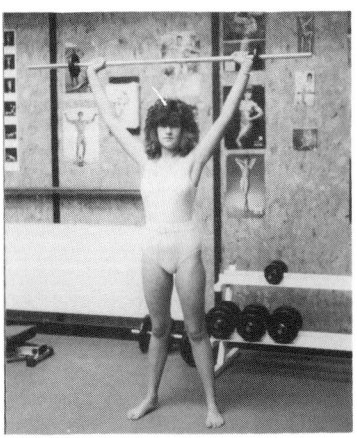

1 *Pick the bar off the floor with a wide grip. Place it behind your neck.*

2 *Press the weight up and lock out your arms. Lower the weight to behind your neck and press again.*

Variation: Upright Rowing

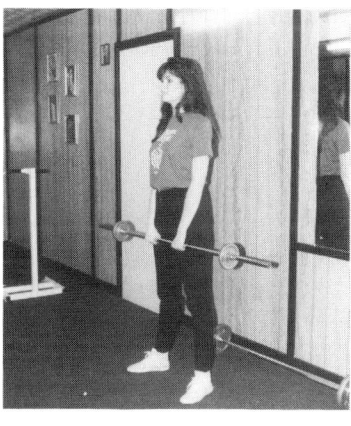 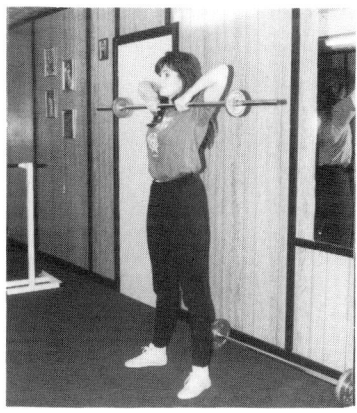

1 *Hold the bar with a narrow grip.*

2 *Pull the bar up to the upper chest keeping it close to the body with the elbows raised.*

Variation: Lateral Raises

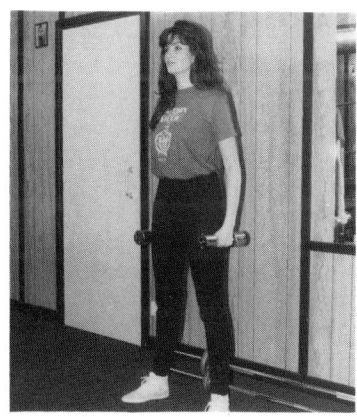 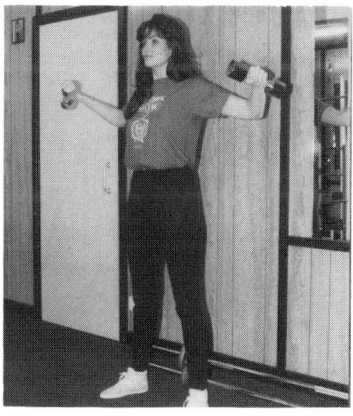

1 *Hold two dumbells in a relaxed standing position.*

2 *Raise the dumbells with your arms slightly bent until they are level with your shoulders, then lower them slowly; repeat the exercise.*

Variation: Bent Over Lateral Raises

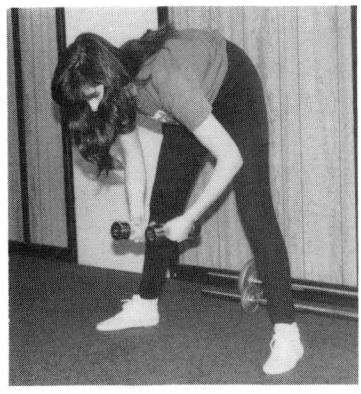 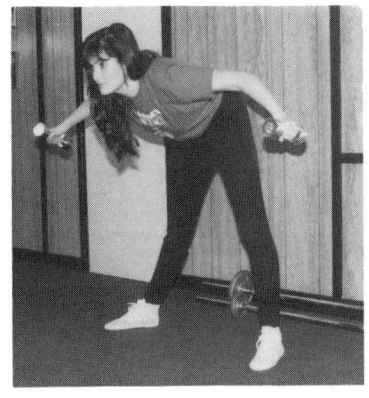

1 *Bend over and take a dumbell in each hand.*

2 *Remaining in the bent position raise the weights together.*

Exercise Four: Triceps (back of upper arm)
Triceps Push-Downs

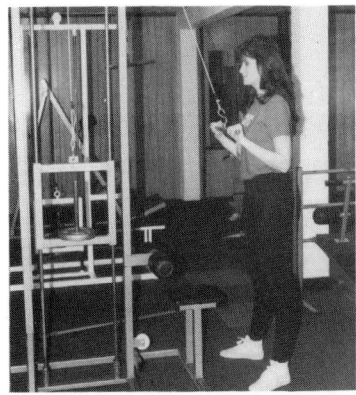 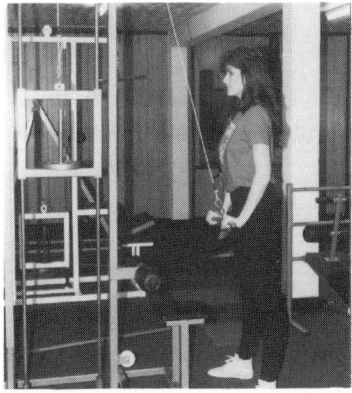

1 *Take the bar of the pulley machine in a narrow grip and hold it at chest level.*

2 *Push down, pivoting at the elbow in a strict movement, moving only the forearms, keeping the upper arm motionless. Elbows should be held in.*

Variation: Lying Tricep Extensions

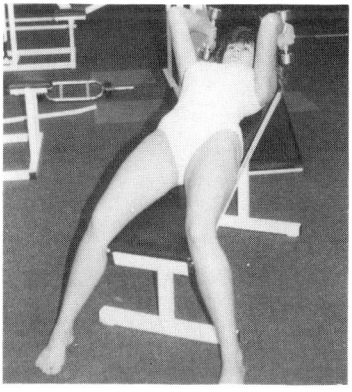 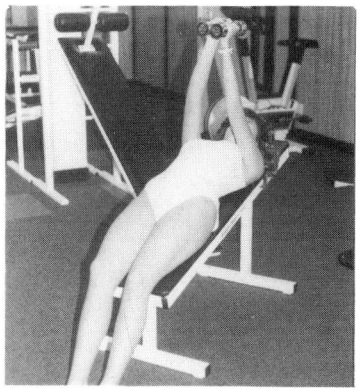

1 *Lie down on the exercise bench and lower the dumbells either side of your forehead, obviously taking care not to hit yourself.*

2 *Raise the weights at the same time, moving only the forearms and keeping your elbows in.*

Variation: Single Arm Tricep Extensions

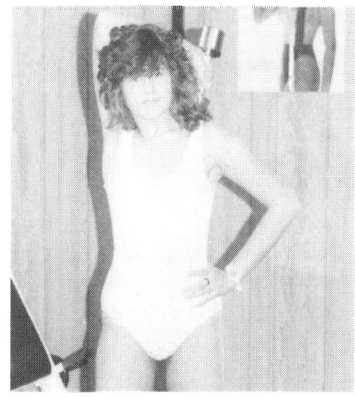 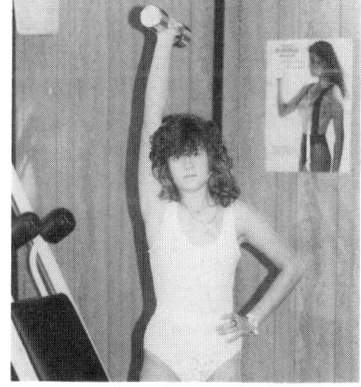

1 *Pick up a dumbell in your right hand and press it over your head letting it fall slowly behind your head. Keep your upper arm close to your head for the whole exercise.*

2 *Straighten the arm, moving the forearm only. Raise and lower the weight for the required number of repetitions and repeat the exercise with the other arm.*

Variation: Standing Tricep Extensions

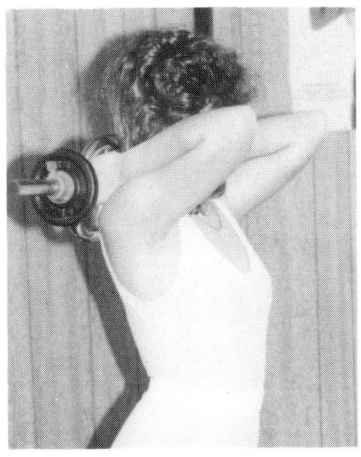 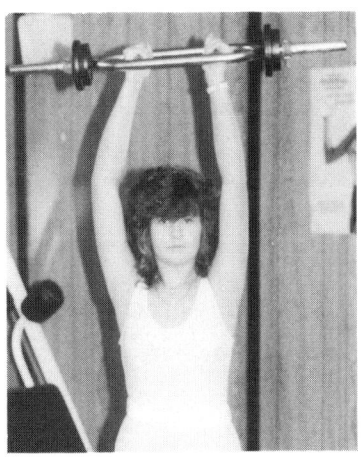

1 *Pick up the bar and lower it behind your head. Keep your elbows in and your upper arms stationary.*

2 *Extend the forearms upwards until the arms are straight. Lower the bar and repeat .*

Exercise Five: Back
Lateral Pull-Downs

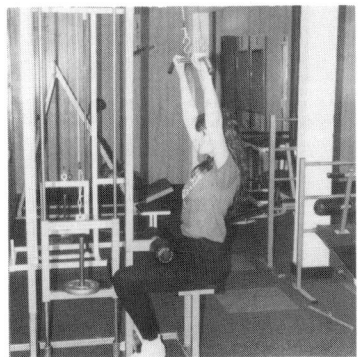 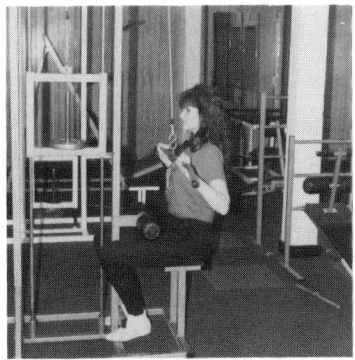

1 *Take hold of the bar of the pulley machine with a wide grip and sit on the seat provided.*

2 *Pull the bar down to your chest. When you let the bar back up, control the weight and let it straighten your arms.*

Variation: Bent-Over Rowing

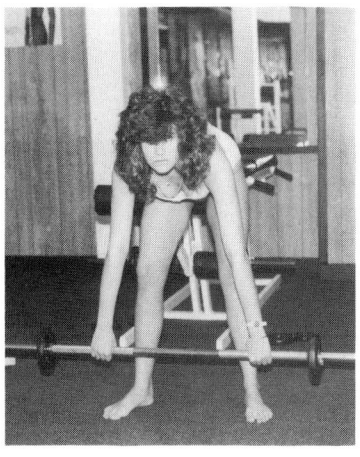 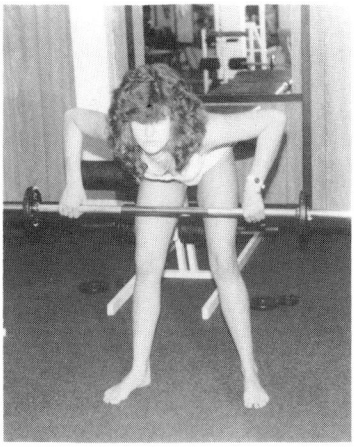

1 *Bend over and pick up the barbell with a grip slightly wider than your shoulders.*

2 *Bend your knees slightly and pull the weight to your stomach. When you lower the weight do not touch the floor.*

Variation: Lower Back Exercise

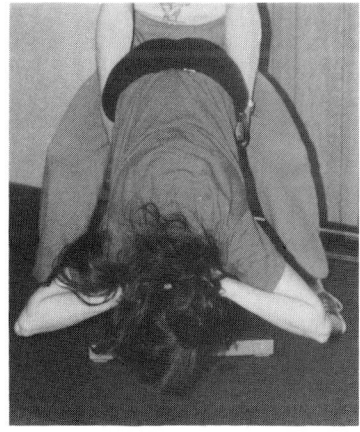 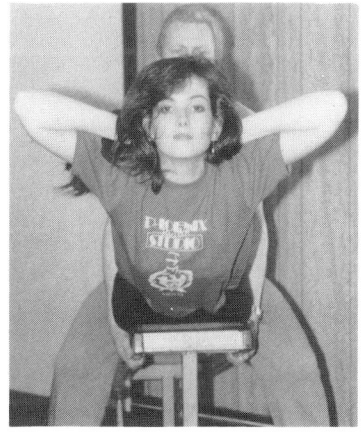

1 *Lie on the incline bench so that with someone sitting on your legs you can dip over the end.*

2 *With your hands behind your head, raise yourself up and down in a slow rhythmic motion.*

Exercise Six: Biceps
Barbell Curl

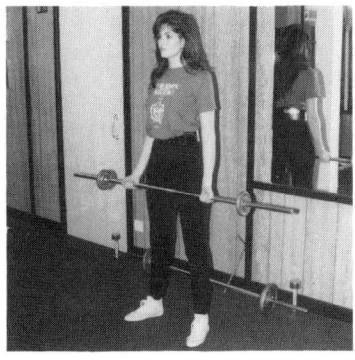 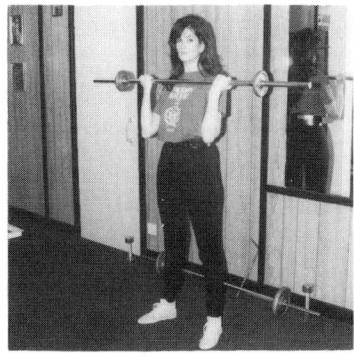

1 *Hold the barbell with a grip just wider than your shoulders and with your palms turned outwards.*

2 *Curl the bar upwards until it is level with your shoulders. Do not swing the weight up but keep the bar close to your body for the full duration of the movement. Lower the barbell slowly to the starting position and repeat.*

Variation: Seated Dumbell Curl

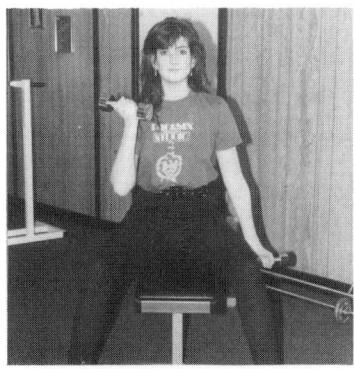 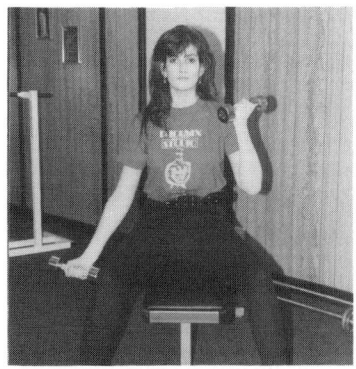

1 *Take two dumbells and sit on an exercise bench. Curl the weight in your right hand.*

2 *Curl the weight in your left hand then repeat alternately with left and right.*

Variation: Concentration Curl

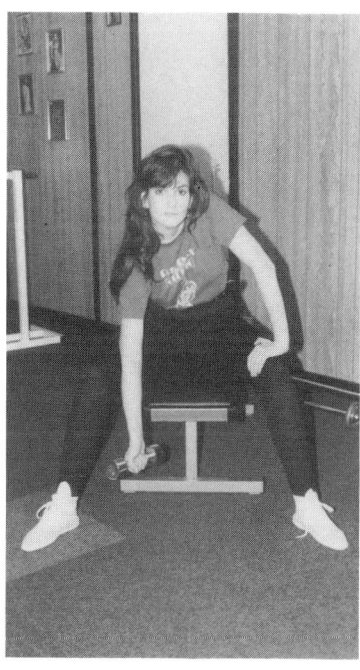

1 *Sit down with a dumbell in your right hand. Put your left hand on your knee for support.*

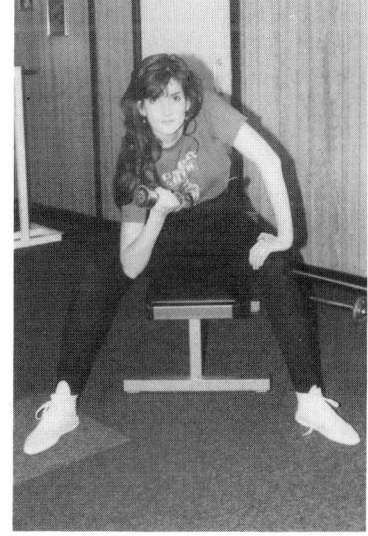

2 *Put your right elbow against the inside of your right knee and curl the weight towards your shoulder.*

Exercise Seven: Waistline (Abdominals)

The waist is so important that all the following exercises should be done at the end of every workout. Incline sit-ups hit the middle abdominals while leg raises hit the lower abdominals. Side bends and twists hit the obliques just above the hips, and crunches hit the upper abdominals.

Incline Situps

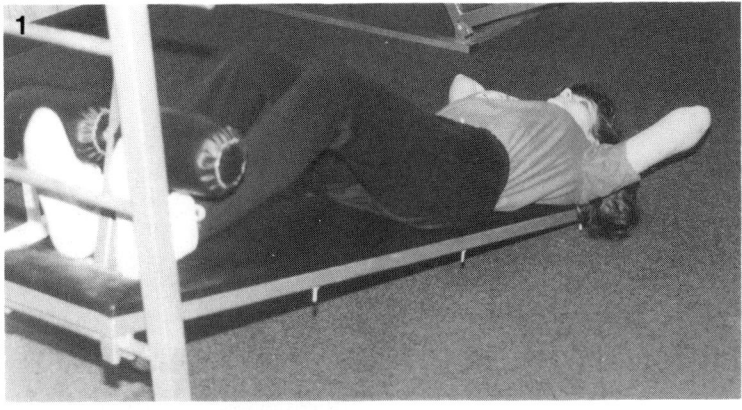

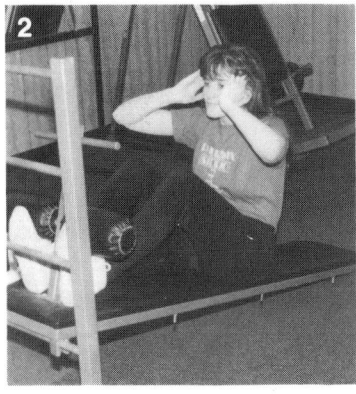

1 *Lie down on the incline board with your toes under the rollers and your knees slightly bent.*

2 *Put your hands by the side of your head and sit up slowly. Lower yourself slowly and immediately repeat the exercise.*

Leg Raises

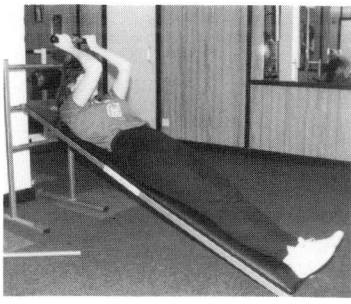 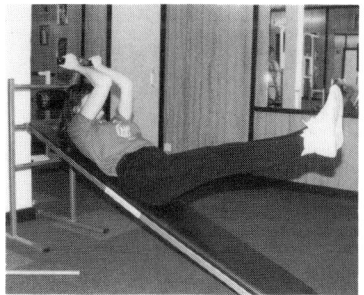

1 *Lie down on the incline board anchoring yourself by holding on to the handle.*

2 *Raise your legs together keeping them straight at all times. Lower them slowly and repeat the exercise.*

Twists

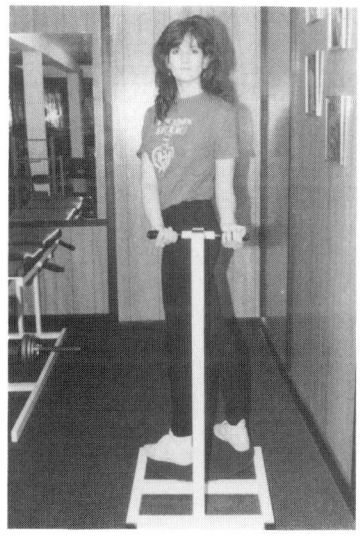 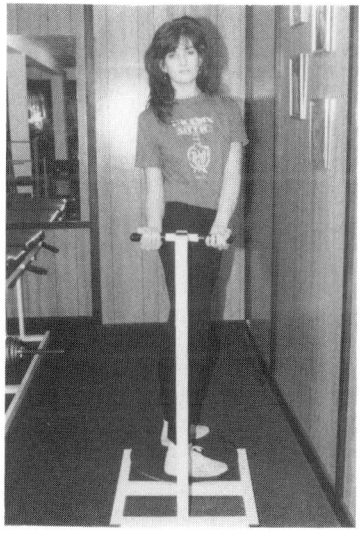

1 *Stand on the free-moving disc and hold on to the handle of the twister. Twist to the right.*

2 *Keeping your shoulders stationary all the time, twist to the left.*

Side Bends

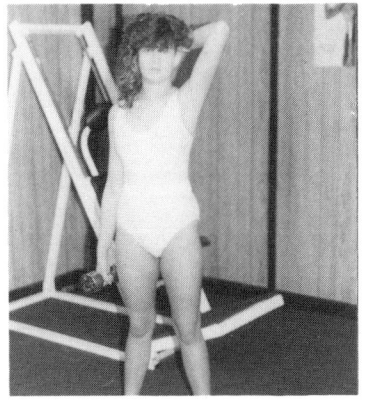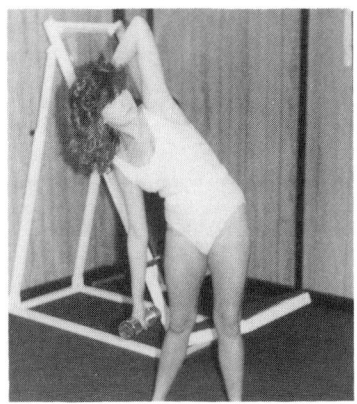

1 *Hold a dumbell at arm's length. Put your free hand behind your head.*

2 *Bend at the waist keeping both your feet flat on the floor, and return to the starting position. Repeat for a number of repetitions before doing the same exercise with the other hand.*

Crunches

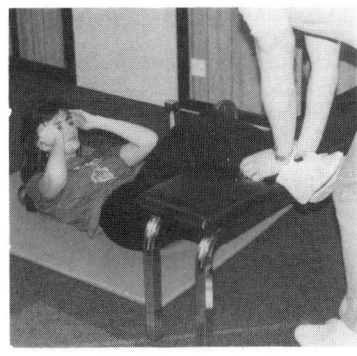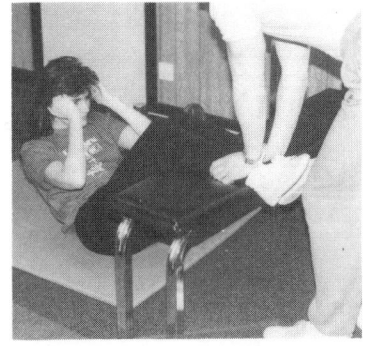

1 *Lie on your back with your feet over the exercise bench. It helps if someone can hold your ankles. Put your hands by your head.*

2 *Raise just your shoulders off the floor. Only half movements are necessary but these should be rapid until you feel a 'burn' in the muscle.*